ST3 Urology national selec... guide

TABLE OF CONTENTS
The structure of the interview 4
The competition……………..5
Competition in 2016 and a planned change in 2017
What to do if you do not score high enough to get a training number?................5
What to do if you think that your interview scores are not fair?....................6
General Advice………………………7
The portfolio station: (max score 64.4)…………..10
Audit ………………………….11
Teaching …………………….12
Volunteer …………………12
Courses in teaching ……….13
What kind of questions you could be asked in the portfolio station?…….13
Common Dos and Don'ts ………….13
Hand-shake ……………13
Prepare your answers early ………………….14
Believe in yourself and don't downplay your achievements…..14
Be enthusiastic and happy ……………………14
Maintain eye contact …………15
Don't let your performance in one station affects your performance in the rest of the stations …...15
Your answers should be brief, concise and interesting……..15
Subscribe to interview preparation courses……..16
Example portfolio questions………………16
The Elective Station………21
How to prepare for this station? …………21
Male LUTS………………….24
Prostate Cancer………37
Bladder cancer……………49
Testicular cancer………..61
Recurrent Urinary Tract Infections………68
Kidney cancer……71

ST3 Urology National Selection Interview Guide
Kass-Iliyya A.

Kidney stones................94
Urinary incontinence..........113
Haematuria......122
Erectile dysfunction..125
The Emergency station..........132
Anaphylaxis....................141
Testicular Torsion......142
Post TURP bleeding...144
TUR syndrome 145
Renal Trauma......147
Infected obstructed kidney.......149
Acute retention of urine 151
Fournier's gangrene...........152
Communication skills............154
The practical skills station........160
Ureteric stenting..........161
Insertion of suprapubic catheter......164
Flexible cystoscopy and TURBT consenting...........166
Circumcision..........169
IV Contrast with renal impairment and Metformin........171
Common Urological procedures BAUS consent forms....171
Appendix....177

ST3   Urology   National   Selection   Interview   Guide
Kass-Iliyya A.

Copyrights and Acknowledgment:

OXFORD HANDBOOK OF UROLOGY by Reynard, Brewster, and Biers (2013)
1,466w and Tab.13.4 from pp.127-146. By permission of Oxford University Press.

Viva Practice for the FRCS(Urol) Examination" by Manit Arya and Iqbal Shergill © 2010 Reproduced by permission of Taylor & Francis Books UK.

ST3 Urology National Selection Interview Guide
Kass-Iliyya A.

Preface:
Why I wrote this book?

I have attended this interview few times before being successful and during my preparation for the Urology national selection interview, I was looking for some guidance and advice, the common "Dos and Don'ts" and how to best invest my time. Unfortunately, I couldn't find many books or resources in this regard.

Most views expressed in this book are my own views, I would advise you to read other sources as appropriate.

As an aspiring urologist, the ST3 urology national selection interview is potentially one of the most important interviews in the life of a urologist in the UK. It is the deciding factor of whether you could progress to specialty training and ultimately practice independently as a consultant. It is not the only way of becoming a consultant but it is the most recognised way and admittedly the most structured way. You are guaranteed decent training and teaching over a period of 5 years, which enables you to gain the experience, skills and knowledge necessary for the award of certificate of completion of training (CCT) in Urology and be admitted on the specialist register and therefore be able to apply for a consultant post in Urology and practice independently. Remember, it is not the only way of becoming a consultant, the CESR route or article 14 is another way which has its own advantages (Staying in one place during training with no need to travel every year for five years, better family life in the initial years, etc....)" See table (8) for a detailed comparison between the two routes in the appendix.

ST3   Urology   National   Selection   Interview   Guide
Kass-Iliyya A.

1. The structure of the interview

The interview is divided into 5 stations. Each station is marked separately,

Station	Mark	Preparation time	Time allocated
Portfolio station	64.4	3 minutes	27 minutes
Elective scenario	32	3 minutes	12 minutes
Emergency scenario	32	3 minutes	12 minutes
Technical skills	32	3 minutes	12 minutes
Communication skills	40	3 minutes	12 minutes
Totals	200	**15 minutes**	**75 minutes**

with some stations having more weight (marks) than others:

Each station will last 12 minutes and you will have 3 minutes to prepare before each station. You will be given a scenario to read during those three minutes and will be provided with a pen and plain paper to write your notes. You are allowed to take your notes inside the station and leave it there at the end. You will hear a bell at the start and end of each station. The portfolio station lasts the longest (12 + 3 + 12) = 27 minutes, **although in the last applicant guide for the 2017 national selection it looks as though this will be reduced to 12 minutes only!**

Please note: you need to score a set minimum of marks to be deemed appointable as a urology ST3. This is usually around 130 marks. This means that you will need to score > 60% to be deemed appointable. If you score less than that you will not be offered any posts. However, being appointable does not automatically mean getting a training number, the latter depends on your rank.
Candidates are ranked based on their interview scores.
Generally speaking, to secure a training number you need to **rank 60** or above and to do so you need to score at least **160-165 marks** out of 200 (80-83%)

4

ST3   Urology   National   Selection   Interview   Guide
Kass-Iliyya A.

The competition:
Usually there are **60 numbers** or so in each round and there are 150-170 candidates, of these; 125-135 or so are usually deemed appointable and 25-45 are deemed non-appointable. So, if you are deemed appointable your chances of getting a number are 30-50% which is reasonable. Having said that, this interview remains highly competitive despite the relatively good chance on paper because the calibre of the candidates is very high. The most high ranking (60 and above) candidates score very closely to each other and ultimately one mark can make a difference between getting a training number or not, so make sure you don't lose any unnecessary marks.

Competition in 2016 and a planned change in 2017:
There were 151 applicants for NTN numbers. 123 were appointable and 64 trainees were appointed. 37% of male applicants (n=23) and 60% of females (n=30) were appointed and 1 indicated no gender preference. 21 (33%) were appointed directly from core training. The next round of National Selection will be held on April 6 and 7, 2017 at Elland Rd Stadium, Leeds. The only planned change **is an updated portfolio station which will be based on models currently in use by most other surgical specialties**. It will rely more on a rigid and detailed scoring system of the applicant's portfolio, and less on a traditional interview format. Applicants will be given clear instructions on what evidence they will be required to show and how they should lay out their portfolios to make scoring as straight forward as possible. We will need more interviewers than previously as each portfolio station will require 4 interviewers rather than 3. Those interviewers who will be at the portfolio station will be briefed in advance on the new format. It is expected that all TPDs will attend the interviews.

What to do if you do not score high enough to get a training number?
Do not be disheartened!
It does not mean that you are not a good urologist. You might be a great urologist or have the potential to become one but:
You did not know how to sell yourself or keep calm under pressure.
You did not prepare enough
You did not practice your answers well enough.
You might be at a slight disadvantage as some of your training or medical school was overseas and your mother tongue is not English.

ST3 Urology National Selection Interview Guide
Kass-Iliyya A.

Lots of overseas-doctors struggle with communication skills as they do not get training in this area as part of their medical school curriculum and the language barrier does not make it any easier.

More importantly **ask for a detailed feedback!**: Under the Freedom of Information Act, you are entitled to a detailed feedback on your interview performance and how the marks were awarded. This is the only way you could find out **why** you were scored low in one given station so that you could address those shortcomings. The standard feedback does not tell you why you were scored as such in each station, whereas the detailed feedback shows you what the interviewers comments were and where you exactly failed. (Example comments: Elective station: needed prompting, Communication skills: did not take responsibility or apologise to patient for the mistake, portfolio: 6 TURPs candidate claimed to have performed but when questioned says was supervised, practical skills: talks more than do) To request a detailed feedback, you would need to make a subject access request, details of which can be found within the FOI (Freedom of information policy) which is available through the (FOI) link at the bottom of the Health Education Yorkshire and Humber Recruitment webpages.

http://www.yorksandhumberdeanery.nhs.uk/recruitment/

Please note that Yorkshire and the Humber deanery FOI are an integral part of Health Education England, as such all requests should be directed via their website

https://www.hee.nhs.uk/about-us/contact-us/freedom-information-act

Once you go on that website they will ask you to submit your query by emailing hee.foia@nhs.net .

Email hee.foia@nhs.net and explain that you are requesting a detailed feedback on your interview performance in the Urology ST3 national selection interview. They usually respond within 6-8 weeks.

What do you do if you think that your interview scores are not fair?

You can raise a complaint. There is a formal complaint procedure on the Yorkshire and the Humber deanery website. You could email the complaint team directly on rec.complaints@yh.hee.nhs.uk alternatively you could email the urology recruitment team and they will direct you on how to do so. Their email is urology.rec@yh.hee.nhs.uk

You need to submit reasonable evidence that supports your claim. If you don't agree with the initial response to your complaint you could appeal against it, but you need to provide further strong evidence to support your appeal otherwise no further action will be taken.

ST3   Urology   National   Selection   Interview   Guide
Kass-Iliyya A.

2. General Advice

Before talking about each station there are general rules one should try and stick to if at all possible.

Preparation

I cannot stress enough the importance of preparation to be able to succeed in this interview. Remember you are competing against very high calibre candidates some of whom have already done PhDs, MDs, and have several publications under their names, let alone ample clinical experience in the specialty.

There is no excuse for not knowing something that you should know. For instance, a question about the bread and butter of urology "male LUTS", you should know this topic thoroughly and in detail. NICE guidelines are a must in this regard. If you fail to answer a question satisfactorily about LUTS and unless you could compensate for that in the other stations, you will probably miss out on a training number because not many people will fail to answer this. Your knowledge level should be set at ST3 level; however, because of the competitive nature of this interview, higher knowledge level is required. Lots of candidates use FRCS urology preparation books (A commonly used book is **viva practice for the FRCS(urol) examination**), which is not unreasonable. A small gap in your knowledge could be the deciding factor for choosing somebody else over you, so aim to close the gaps in your knowledge as much as possible. The interview is not the time to scratch your head and think about the answers, it's the time to shine and confidently deliver your previously prepared and rehearsed answers. Interviewers could easily tell the difference between a candidate who is well prepared and another who is not.

Preparation applies to all 5 stations, you cannot be prepared enough so keep preparing closer to the day of the interview. I will talk about how to prepare in more detail in each section. An excellent way to prepare for the knowledge station is to sit with your consultant and do a work based assessment like Mini-CEX or CBD, afterwards you will know the gaps and weaknesses in your knowledge and you will have the chance to correct those. Choose a consultant who likes to drill his registrars! Remember, prepare equally for all the stations, don't focus only on one area and ignore other areas (a common mistake).

Know your strengths and weaknesses and do not ignore the latter

The worst mistake that you could make is to ignore your areas of weaknesses and hope that you will not be tested in those areas. Do not leave anything to luck. We all have a tendency to read more about subjects that are of interest to us and ignore the subjects that we don't like. However, in the interview you could be asked about anything that is appropriate for ST3 level and this includes a huge range of subjects. The best way of knowing your weaknesses is to choose a subject and pretend that you are teaching medical students or junior doctors about it, and ask yourself questions that students could be asking you as you start talking about the subject and see whether you could answer those questions satisfactorily. For instance, medical treatment options for male LUTS include Tamsulosin, Finasteride, or a combination of the two +_ anticholinergics depending on the symptoms, but not all of us know when to give Tamsulosin alone, when to give finasteride alone, when to give a combination of the two and when to add an anti-cholinergic. If you read NICE guidelines about male LUTS you could easily answer those questions. Another typical example is "communication skills", an area that lots of doctors struggle with, due to different reasons, and therefore ignoring it instead of practicing with a work colleague or even with a family member or a friend is another big mistake.

Enjoy the interview

I came to realise the importance of this advice quite late in the process after I attended the interview several times. It sounds silly when you hear it first and I used to brush this advice off thinking "how can you enjoy something that you fear". However, it's golden advice, **with the proviso** that you prepare well. if you prepare well for the interview, you'll confidently showcase your knowledge and skills. Even the interviewers will enjoy listening to you. Remember people go to theatres and musicals to watch or listen to very well prepared actors or musicians and they enjoy the experience, thanks to the very hard work that those actors or musicians put into making the experience such a success. Equally actors and musicians also enjoy seeing the crowds in awe listening to their hard work. Nobody wants to listen to an ill prepared actor or musician who gets his notes wrong! So, if you are not well prepared you will not be able to enjoy the interview and simply there will be no harvest to reap.

Prepare well in advance

ST3 Urology National Selection Interview Guide
Kass-Iliyya A.

This is not an ordinary interview that you prepare for in a week or so and hope for the best. This is a life-changing interview and the competition is strong. Therefore, preparation should start well in advance of the interview to be able to stand out on the day. Think of the interview as an exam rather than an interview. In my personal estimation, you need 4-6 months to prepare fully for the interview and obviously the more you prepare the better your chances will be. Remember good preparation reduces the stress of the interview, reduces your fear of certain questions or topics, increases your confidence, allows you to enjoy the interview and boosts your chances of securing a training number (a win-win situation).

Familiarise yourself with the interview:

Imagine yourself driving on a new unfamiliar road. It will take you some time to get used to the road. You will drive slower than usual and you will feel stressed deciding which lane or which turn to take. Other drivers familiar with the road will drive faster, more confidently and they will feel less stressed because they know what is coming ahead and what they should do. It is the same with the interview, familiarise yourself with the structure of the interview and prepare for each station in advance. (I hope this book helps you achieve that) to reduce the chances of any surprises on the day and boost your confidence.

3. The portfolio station: (max score 64.4)

This is very important station and needless to say has the highest marks; (64.4) marks out of (200) total marks. There are several points that the interviewers are looking for:

CV/Career progression

Degree certificates, evidence of completion of MRCS, Foundation and Core competencies. Including Core training certificates with details of jobs undertaken for UK graduates and for others certificates of completion of posts from their trainers, programme directors or equivalent,

Course completion certificates,

Evidence of Prizes awarded.

Copies of the audits plus signed certification from trainers if presented or copy of journal / acceptance letter from journal if published,

Details and evidence of Teaching Experience

Copies of posters / presentations certified by trainers with details of where presented. Copies of Publications or letters of acceptance from peer reviewed journals for all publications.

Log book (this should not contain easily identifiable patient details other than unit number and date of birth or age) All these points are equally important.

As alluded to earlier there are plans to change the structure of this station in 2017 to better reflect the substance and the contents of the candidate's portfolio rather than his/her ability to answer different interview questions.

As a CT2 doctor (**Third of the total NTN went to core trainees in 2016**) you have a very good chance of scoring high on the career progression as there are no years worked as trust grade/specialty doctor. However, most core trainees lack on the other aspects of the portfolio like publications and clinical experience due to their limited time in the specialty. Having said that, too much experience counts against the candidate's score as there is a weighting system which means that if you spent many years as a trust grade/specialty doctor or even LAT ST3, the time you spent will be taken into account when determining your portfolio station score to make it fair play, because needless to say if you spend more time as a urology SpR you are likely to have a better logbook and more academic achievements. Therefore, if you have more than 12 months as an SpR in Urology your score will be weighted by 1.15. (an example of a score breakdown is included in Figure (1)).

Station	Your Score	Maximum Score
Portfolio (includes a weighting of 1.15)	51.75	64.4
Scenario Out-Patient	32	32
Scenario Emergency	30	32
Communication	18	40
Skills	27	32
TOTAL	158.75	200.4

Figure (1): Score breakdown after a Urology ST3 national selection interview (Trainee ranked 63 and was offered a LAT job after this interview, an example of how poor score in one station (communication skills in this case) could result in losing out on a training number)

Audit:
It's never too late to do an audit and close the loop, it doesn't have to be a big audit, for example 20 patients will suffice. You could pick something that you could do over the computer without having to pull all the patients notes. If you are working with a keen FY1 or CT1 they could be of great help. The first step after having an audit idea is to register your audit

with the audit department at your local hospital so that you could make it official and get a certificate of proof after finalising and presenting your results. An example audit is the appropriateness of the initial investigations of patients presenting with acute renal colic. You could rely on BAUS recommendation and compare the hospital protocol or practice with those. A common shortfall is forgetting to check calcium and uric acid levels for those patients and after identifying such shortcomings you could recommend changing the order set in A/E to include those tests.

Make sure your logbook is up to date and be aware of putting inaccurate information on it.

For example, in one of my interviews I had 45 TURPs at the time and I put 6 performed, although I did all six from start to finish by myself, I was supervised by consultants in all of them. However, the fact that I put performed gave the impression that I did all six by myself without any supervision, when I was asked about this I had to clarify and said: **'sorry I made a mistake I should have put supervised instead of performed'** and the interviewer was not completely satisfied with that which reflected negatively on my score and feedback. So, make sure you put accurate accounts of your role in each operation and make sure all of them are supervised, as you are not supposed to do any operation unsupervised at an ST3 level except perhaps flexible cystoscopies. Interviewers will pick up on that and it might raise safety and probity issues even if it was a simple recording mistake.

Teaching:
Evidence (Feedback forms):
If you deliver any teaching for medical students, nurses or junior doctors on the ward, make sure you always have feedback forms ready to handout, as these will be your main proof of teaching delivery. It's also useful to plan for teaching in advance and prepare power-point slides with the date of the teaching and the subject on the first slide. This will serve as another proof that you have actually delivered the teaching. Some people go to extra lengths and take pictures of themselves and the audience during deliverance and include it in the portfolio. Whatever you do, make sure your teaching is interesting, interactive, and problem based so that you could get good feedback. It is also worth aiming to deliver teaching to larger groups (20 or more pupils) as this will be weightier and will show confidence and good ability of public speaking. Furthermore, you could get a certificate at the end of the teaching session from the relevant institution.

Volunteer

You could volunteer to deliver teaching to medical students by emailing the post-graduate centre teaching coordinator and say that you are interested in delivering teaching in Urology to large groups. Volunteering demonstrates that you show initiative and you could use it as an example in the portfolio station as a measure you have undertaken to enhance your personal development and subsequently your training. Some hospitals also do grand-rounds where a controversial topic is selected and you could volunteer to present that topic yourself. Usually this is presented to the whole department including junior as well as senior doctors and it serves as an excellent example of taking the initiative.

Courses in teaching

Make sure you attend "**Teach the Teacher**" course by Oxford Medical.

What kind of questions could you be asked in the portfolio station?

This could be anything from CV questions to hobbies and pastimes.

Take us through your CV
What are your strengths and weaknesses?
Describe a bad day and a good day at work
How do you de-stress or deal with stress?
Where do you see yourself in 5 or 10 years' time?
Give an example where you took the initiative in the last 2 weeks
What did you do to enhance your training?
How do you stand out from the crowd?
What are your proudest achievements (career and also personal) and why?
Talk us through a mistake that you made, how you rectified it and what did you learn from it?
What do you think of research? Should every doctor do research
Why you chose urology?
Give an example of leadership, team work
What are your hobbies, what do you enjoy doing?
What do you think of your career progression so far? Or your training so far?
Give us an example of an audit you did and what did you learn from it? Did you close the loop?
Talk us through your teaching experience
Questions about the NHS (not commonly asked)
How do you convince a commissioning group to fund a robot in your department where a laparoscopic surgery is currently the main used technique?

Tell me about any patient feedback you have received.
Obviously you need to sit down and answer each of these 20 questions according to your situation.

Common Dos and Don'ts

Hand-shake:
This is a tricky area and there are no fast rules, you will often know what to do on the day, however, as a general rule: only shake the interviewers' hands if they offer to do so. I wouldn't necessarily volunteer to shake the interviewers' hands especially if they do not seem to be willing to do so, or if you are far away from them. (i.e. separated by a table)

Prepare your answers early:
Don't leave it to the interview day to answer those questions, even if you worked them out in your mind. You need to practice what you are going to say and say it out loud in front of your spouse, relative, a mirror or a video-recorder. Ask for feedback or watch yourself afterwards and criticize yourself. You will probably look shaky, weak and hesitant at first but after a few times, it will become second nature to you and you will be able to deliver your answers smoothly and confidently. This will make all the difference between someone who is prepared and someone who is not. Your delivery is extremely important and the interviewers are looking for a confident self-assured registrar who knows him or herself well and knows their strengths and weaknesses. Someone who is mature enough and could be trusted to take responsibility.

Believe in yourself and don't downplay your achievements.
This is a classic mistake as well. Sadly, lots of people lack confidence and tend to under-estimate themselves and their achievements. **If you don't believe in yourself no one will**. There is no point in going to the interview if you deep down think that you stand no chance and that others are much better than yourself. You need to always focus on your strengths when you answer any question and showcase that strength with confident delivery. Even if you do not think the audit you did is important, the chances are it highlighted some deficiencies in the system which you could focus on with a positive tone. Remember **defeatist attitude** means that you admit defeat. This means you set yourself for failure and deny yourself any chance of success right from the start. However, if you feel defeated and lack in confidence, maybe you should examine yourself again, probe deeper and ask yourself: **is this really what I am passionate about and what I want to do?** If you are passionate about something you should not feel defeated, on the contrary you should feel that you are the

best in the field and be very confident. Otherwise, think twice about taking a career in Urology.

Be enthusiastic and happy
I personally fell for this trap a few times, in fact it cost me a research registrar job at a big tertiary centre in a previous interview where the feedback was: "got all the essential and desirable personal specification but not enthusiastic and convincing enough". With the heat of the interview and after perhaps underperforming in the previous station or due to personal circumstances, we sometimes feel despondent or a bit low in mood. This will give the wrong impression of de-motivation. No one would like to interview a de-motivated registrar who couldn't wait for this interview to finish; the interviewers will feel that they are wasting their time with someone who is not even interested in the job! Look happy and very interested but equally don't crack jokes and overdo it.

Maintain eye contact
Maintaining eye contact is a sign of confidence, good communication and inter-personal skills. It shows that you are a mature and brave registrar who is willing to address issues face to face and take responsibility. It also shows a lot of respect to interviewers who took the trouble to come and interview you and would expect you to acknowledge their presence and at least look them in the eye. Also remember to look at all the interviewers during the portfolio station and not only focus on the person who is asking you the questions as others might feel ignored and marginalised during the interview which they might interpret as a lack of respect even if it was not intended.

Don't let your performance in one station affect your performance in the rest of the stations.
Another classical mistake, if you think you didn't do well in one station; don't let it ruin your chances in the other stations. Remember these points:
It might not be as bad as you think.
All the other candidates might have not fared well in this station
One mark could be the deciding factor for getting a number or not so don't ruin your chances by adopting the wrong attitude and losing unnecessary marks in the next station.

Your answers should be brief, concise and interesting.
Do not talk for more than 2 minutes at the maximum when answering a certain question. Most interviewers lose interest in your answer if it's too long and lacks structure. You need to score as many points as possible in the little time available. Aim to showcase your strengths in each answer. A

great way of answering questions is to signpost your answers and to give a summary at the beginning. For instance, if you were asked "why you chose a career in urology?" Your answer could be something like: "I chose a career in urology for three main reasons

Clinically: I enjoy the mix of medicine and surgery and working in the operating theatre environment

Academically: great potential for research and academic career

Personally: great lifestyle and family friendly specialty"

By doing this you will grab the attention of the interviewers, you will look well prepared and you will score maximum points.

Subscribe to interview preparation courses:

There are plenty of very good interview preparation courses which will focus on the points mentioned above and help you identify your weaknesses so that you are better equipped to pass this interview. (I personally found ISC medical ST3 preparation course very helpful, other candidates choose the Hammersmith interview course). They are certainly worth the money.

3.1. Example portfolio questions:

Talk us through your cv?

This is a very common question and usually is the first question that you will be asked in the portfolio station. This could be a bit tedious but you could make it really interesting by focusing on the relevant points to a career in urology which is what the interviewers are looking for, otherwise nobody would like to listen to detailed accounts of your non-surgical rotations as such information is irrelevant to this interview.

For example, I graduated from xxxx University and did my foundation training in the xxxx deanery, I rotated in OBG, breast surgery, acute medicine and urology and I enjoyed the surgical specialties the most, therefore I applied for a core surgical training which I did in the xxxx deanery. During my core training I did an MSc in surgical sciences at the university of xxxx this was culminated with a dissertation where I passed with distinction, the topic of which was urological, I also published my dissertation in a peer reviewed journal. Urology stood out for me in all the surgical specialties and I started my specialty training as a LAT in the xxxx region. My first job was a great introduction to general and core urology where I learned to perform both rigid and flexible cystoscopies under supervision as well as small TURPs and TURBTs. My subsequent rotation was in a renowned cancer centre in xxxx where I was involved in complicated cancer surgeries, and from thereon I did an academic research job in xxxx where I was the main coordinator of a randomised feasibility study comparing two surgical treatments for male stress incontinence after prostatectomy. I was also involved in several research projects at the time, all of which culminated with national and international presentation as well as peer reviewed publications. I won the best paper prize at xxxx, where following from that I did a trust grade job for a year in xxxx and currently am doing a LAT ST3 job in xxxx deanery. I have been exposed to a wide breadth of urological procedures and I am confident in performing all the common urological emergencies, including scrotal exploration, insertion of a JJ stent, insertion of difficult urethral catheters including suprapubic catheters. I feel that I am ready and very well equipped to enter the specialty-training programme and I am very excited to be able to offer a lot and learn a lot simultaneously.

What are your strengths and weaknesses?

The **CAMP** structure is a life-saver when it comes to the urology ST3 interview, virtually all the answers revolve around this structure in one way or another.

C Clinically
A Academically
M Management
P Personal

So when you are asked about your strengths, think CAMP immediately.

Clinically: What can you do and at what level of competence? (be honest and do not oversell yourself, otherwise you will come across as someone who wouldn't really benefit from the training programme as you already had the skills and the knowledge).

Academically: publications, presentations, awards, degrees.

Management: rota coordination, managing juniors, doing a management course, etc....

Personally: team player (you need to give an example very briefly), good communicator (I have received a lot of positive feedback about my communication skills and about my sensitive and understanding approach to patients when breaking bad news).

When it comes to weaknesses, the golden rule is "avoid weaknesses that could be misinterpreted as a sign of unsafety or could have negative consequences on your firm". The safest two options are:

Difficulty delegating: I find it **hard to delegate** sometimes (because I worry that the job will not be done which might be detrimental to patients) this can cost me some extra time to finish my daily work and can impact my family and social life.

How do you deal with it? I get to know my juniors better and establish a relationship of trust. Regularly teach the juniors about urology to make sure they understand what I delegate to them. (This shows a lot of insight and management skills)

Too enthusiastic: I find myself **agreeing to take on too many projects** at the same time (because I am very enthusiastic and I like to achieve) although I always deliver on time, this sometimes can take away from my social and family time and cause me some added stress. (Remember as long as it doesn't affect your productivity at work, this is not really a bad weakness. At the end of the day not seeing your family as often as you'd like is a personal cost but it's not going to affect your firm)

How to deal with it? Learn to match the number of projects I agree to take on with the available time, to avoid stress and impact on family life, also learn to say no when you think that you will not be able to achieve.

Where do you see yourself in 5 or 10 years' time?
An example answer:
(Remember the **CAMP** structure again).
I see myself as a consultant urologist working in a teaching hospital. Clinically: I would like to specialise in oncology and I would aspire to perform robotic prostate surgery, something that I immensely enjoy and love to excel in. Academically: I would like to enhance my academic profile and get involved in research and clinical trials and working in a teaching centre will help me achieve my academic aspirations. In terms of management I would like to set up a special clinic to manage incontinence and erectile dysfunction following prostate surgery. And finally, personally I see myself working in the xxxx deanery due to my personal family ties.

What are your proudest achievements?
(Again, use the **CAMP** structure)
Clinically: I am able to perform all the emergency urological procedures independently, including scrotal exploration, insertion of JJ stent, inserting of difficult urethral catheter using flexible cystoscopy and guide-wire and insertion of suprapubic catheter.
Academically: I passed my MSc degree with distinction from the university of xxxx and I published my dissertation in a peer review journal, this gave me huge confidence in my academic skills including literature review,

critical appraisal and writing a paper, I also won the best paper prize at xxxx where I competed against a very high calibre academic work which gave me a big drive to believe in myself and continue to excel.

Personally: I got married and I have a child.

Talk us through a mistake that you made how you rectified it and what did you learn?

This is another tricky question. The key here is not to mention a mistake that resulted in harm to patients.

Common examples are:

Prescription errors which did not result in harm.

Rare side effect of a medication: for example an Oculogyric crisis (dystonic reaction) after giving an anti-emetic to a patient post-operatively.

Consenting the wrong patient with the same name and realising the mistake very early on in the process. The key here is to realise the mistake, correct it, apologise to the patient and reflect/learn from it and make sure it doesn't happen again.

Giving trimethoprim to a patient on methotrexate. This increases the risk of bone marrow depression and other haematological toxicities. An example scenario:

A patient who is coming for ESWL lithotripsy had e-coli positive urine culture, and the nurse informed you that the culture results are back and its sensitive to Trimethoprim. You checked the allergies on the system and prescribed her a 5 day course of Trimethoprim and requested the notes. When the notes arrived the next day you realised that the patient takes Methotrexate for Rheumatoid arthritis, you identified the mistake immediately and you phoned the patient and asked her to stop taking the Trimethoprim immediately. You phoned the haematology registrar for advice and he advised you to monitor the patient's blood and administer IV folinic acid if there are any signs of bone marrow suppression. In this case the patient was very well, her bloods were normal, she was on a small dose of Methotrexate and she only took two tables of Trimethoprim before realising this mistake. No harm came to the patient and she did not require any treatment. My action: I apologised to patient, I asked her to come to hospital to check her bloods, I contacted haematology for advice. What did I learn?

Always check drug interactions as well as allergies before prescribing any medications.

Have the patient's notes before prescribing antibiotics to be able to have the full picture.

ST3   Urology   National   Selection   Interview   Guide
Kass-Iliyya A.

What do you think of research? Should everybody be doing research?
This is one of those questions where there is no right or wrong answer. As long as your answer is balanced and you could justify it then you are doing ok.
This is an example answer: I think research is very important to advance the current knowledge, have a better understanding of common diseases and discover new treatments. I believe every doctor should have an exposure to a research environment to enable him/her to better understand and interpret the available evidence and be able to apply it in his or her practice. This could be achieved regionally and nationally via getting involved in national clinical trials, research labs, visiting centres of excellence or locally via setting up journal clubs, or doing a research project relying on the available patients' data at the local hospital. It's important for every doctor to understand the levels of evidence and critically appraise research outcomes and papers and also have some understanding of the setting up and running of clinical trials. Having said that I don't believe that everybody should be doing a **research degree** like MD or PhD, as this will require a lot of determination and enthusiasm over two to three years, the ability to apply for research grants and persevere, and the ability to deal with negative or disappointing findings. I believe that whoever is doing a research degree should have the right mind-set to stay the course, otherwise a lot of energy and resources will be wasted and the whole experience might become negative and regrettable.
So in a nutshell: every doctor should be involved in research but not every doctor should be doing a research degree.

Why you chose urology?
You need to use the **CAMP** technique here as I alluded to earlier.
Clinically: mention what you enjoy the most about working in urology and why. Combination of surgery and medicine, enjoy team work in operating theatre, enjoy operating and theatre environment more than the wards, treating different age groups and gender, involves major as well as minor surgeries which gives lots of career options, dealing with sensitive issues that require excellent communication skills, urology at forefront of cutting edge technology/ robotic surgery. The reasons are endless....
Academically: huge potential for research in areas like prostate cancer and functional urology.
Personally: life-style, compared to other surgical specialties it is family friendly (I wouldn't stress the life-style point too much as this might give the wrong impression that you are prioritising your life-style over your

work which is - although sensible - not usually taken as a sign of being motivated/career driven by the interviewers).

4. The Elective Station

The elective station is usually based on an outpatient scenario.
Possible scenarios include (This is not exclusive)
Male LUTS
Recurrent UTIs
Haematuria
Bladder/Kidney/Prostate/Testicular cancer
Raised PSA
Testicular lump
Renal mass on USS
Haematuria as above.
Incontinence

Possible topics: **Erectile dysfunction, Infertility**, although these topics are thought to be very specialised.

Losing marks in this station is unforgiving, because this is purely a knowledge based station and losing marks can only mean that you are not prepared enough and have not done your homework. If you do lose marks you will be disadvantaged compared to other candidates who are better prepared. This station usually tests your generic knowledge in the context of an outpatient urology clinic addressing common topics, which a urologist encounters on a daily basis. There is always an element of communication skills in this station as well as the emergency station, where the candidate is given a scenario that involves breaking bad news to patients or answering to an angry relative because of a delayed investigation and diagnosis or communicating the need of an anaesthetic assessment (C-PEX cardio-pulmonary exercise testing) and the risk of a general anaesthetic to an elderly patient who has a stag-horn calculus and is considering PCNL. Or going through the consent form with a patient who is due to have an orchidectomy for a suspected testicular cancer including discussion around sperm banking and an insertion of a prosthesis and a biopsy of the other testicle.

How to prepare for this station?
This is very simple. Again there are general rules:

Guidelines

NICE guidelines: You need to know NICE guidelines - which most urologists in the UK follow and adhere to - by heart.
To access follow the link:
https://www.nice.org.uk/guidance/conditions-and-diseases/urological-conditions
Remember if you were asked about something in the NICE guidelines and you didn't know it, then you are running a high risk of losing out on a training number as others will have prepared better and will answer better.
These cover the following areas
Bladder cancer
Lower urinary tract symptoms
Penile and testicular cancer
Prostate cancer
Urinary incontinence

EAU Guidelines
To access follow the link:
http://uroweb.org/guidelines/

BAUS Guidelines (British Association of Urological Surgeons)
To access follow the link:
http://www.baus.org.uk/professionals/baus_business/publications/archive?page=1
These include:
Haematuria guidelines (now withdrawn)
Chronic pelvic pain guidelines
Transrectal ultrasound and prostatic biopsy (very useful guide)
BAUS Suprapubic catheter practice guidelines
Bladder cancer MDT
Briefing paper on biomarkers
Diagnosis of LUTS resulting from BPH (very useful article)
Flexible cystoscopy guidelines

Prostate cancer MDT (Excellent guide to managing prostate cancer)
Renal cancer MDT
Stone Guidelines
Urinary incontinence

Books:

Viva practice for the FRCS urology

https://www.amazon.co.uk/Viva-Practice-FRCS-Examination-MasterPass

You need to read this book from cover to cover more than once. You could potentially skip paediatric urology as it is very specialised topic if you don't have enough time. But again everything is possible.

Oxford handbook of urology

https://www.amazon.co.uk/Handbook-Urology-Flexicover-Medical-Handbooks

Also an invaluable read and a must for all UK urologists (many UK urologists call it the scaffolding that you need to build your knowledge on).

4.1. Male LUTS

History
LUTS History
Voiding symptoms
Storage symptoms
Onset, duration, severity, **impact/troublesome** nature
Incontinence (stress, urge), Nocturia
Ask specifically about
Bedwetting (HPCR)
Storage symptoms and bladder pain (CIS)
Visible haematuria (Bladder, Kidney ca, stones)
Back pain, Neurological symptoms (prostate ca, neuropathic bladder)
Lifestyle
Fluid intake
Adjustments tried by patient
Bowel function red flags (change of bowel habit, weight loss, rectal bleeding, family history of bowel ca)
Sexual function (very important as any intervention or medication can affect the sexual function and can be devastating to a patient, so this should be explored very early on in the consultation. For example: Tamsulosin and TURP can cause retrograde ejaculation and TURP can cause erectile dysfunction)
General: Anorexia, weight loss, tiredness, leg swelling.
If female **obstetrics and gynaecological history**

Smoking History
Occupational History
Travel History
Surgical History
urethral injury/instrumentation
pelvic surgery
Radiotherapy
Medical History
Diabetes
HTN
Neurological disease (Parkinson, MS)
Family History
Urological cancer
Medication History
Diuretics
Sympathomimetic and anticholinergics
Observation
Fluid overload, signs of uraemia
Tremor, gait disturbance
Visible full bladder
Examination
Abdomen (palpable bladder, ballotable kidney)
Enlarged kidneys
Genitals testicle, penis (phymosis, meatal stenosis)
DRE (prostate size, consistency, nodules)
Neurological exam (perianal sensation) (anal tone and sensation)

Questionnaires
IPSS
8 items questionnaire, 7 urinary symptoms, one quality of life (0-7, 8-19, 20-35)
FVC (Polyuria, nocturnal polyuria)
Recommended mandatory Tests
Urinalysis (blood, glucose, protein, leucocytes, nitrites)
Serum creatinine and eGFR **if** suspected renal impairment.
PSA **if** LUTS suggestive of BOO/BPE, abnormal feeling prostate, pt concerned. (See NICE guidelines below)
Flow rate, post void residual (PVR) measurement
Optional tests
USS KUB

If creatinine is high or
Loin pain
Haematuria
Renal enlargement or mass on exam
Cystoscopy
if history of
Haematuria
Equivocal flow rate
Previous Urological surgery
TRUS
Indications:
High PSA
Abnormal DRE
Surgical planning
Urodynamic before surgical intervention
Indication:
Equivocal flow rates VV < 150, Q max >10 ml
Age <50 >80
Previous unsuccessful treatment for BPH
Neurological disease
I include here a summary of NICE guidelines for male LUTS
NICE Guidelines LUTS
Assessment (GP assessment):
Offer:
An assessment of general medical history to identify possible causes and co-morbidities, including
a review of all current medication (including herbal and over-the-counter medication) that may be contributing to the problem.
A physical examination guided by symptoms and other medical conditions,
Examination of the abdomen
Examination of external genitalia
Digital rectal examination
A urine dipstick test to detect blood, glucose, protein, leucocytes and nitrites.
Ask patients with bothersome lower urinary tract symptoms to complete a **urinary frequency volume chart**.
Offer a serum creatinine test (plus estimated glomerular filtration rate calculation) only if you suspect renal impairment:
Palpable bladder,

Nocturnal enuresis,
Recurrent urinary tract infections
History of renal stones

For patients whose lower urinary tract symptoms are not bothersome or complicated,
Give reassurance,
Offer advice on lifestyle interventions (for example, fluid intake) and information on their condition.
Offer review if symptoms change.

For patients with mild or moderate bothersome lower urinary tract symptoms,
Discuss active surveillance (reassurance and lifestyle advice without immediate treatment and with regular follow-up) or
Active intervention (conservative management, drug treatment or surgery).
Offer patients considering treatment for lower urinary tract symptoms an assessment of their baseline symptoms with a validated symptom score (for example, the International Prostate Symptom Score).

PSA testing
Offer patients information, advice and time to decide if they wish to have PSA testing if:
Their lower urinary tract symptoms are suggestive of bladder outlet obstruction secondary to benign prostate enlargement or
Their prostate feels abnormal on digital rectal examination or
They are concerned about prostate cancer (manage suspected prostate cancer in line with the NICE pathways on prostate cancer and suspected cancer recognition and referral).

Tests that should not be offered routinely
Do not routinely offer:
Cystoscopy to patients with no evidence of bladder abnormality
Imaging of the upper urinary tract to patients with no evidence of bladder abnormality (uncomplicated LUTS)
Flow-rate measurement
Post-void residual volume measurement.

Conservative management

Storage symptoms
If you suspect overactive bladder, offer
Supervised bladder training,
Advice on fluid intake,
Lifestyle advice and, if needed,
Containment products.
Offer supervised pelvic floor muscle training to men with stress urinary incontinence caused by prostatectomy.
Advise patients to continue the exercises for at least 3 months before considering other options.
Do not offer penile clamps.

Containment products
For patients with storage lower urinary tract symptoms (particularly urinary incontinence):
offer temporary containment products (for example, pads or collecting devices) to achieve social continence until a diagnosis and management plan have been discussed
offer a choice of containment products based on individual circumstances and in consultation with the patient.
offer external collecting devices (sheath appliances, pubic pressure urinals) before considering indwelling catheterisation (see long-term catheterisation and containment in this pathway).
provide containment products at point of need, and advice about relevant support groups.

Voiding symptoms
Offer intermittent bladder catheterisation before indwelling urethral or suprapubic catheterisation if lower urinary tract symptoms cannot be corrected by less invasive measures.
Tell patients with proven bladder outlet obstruction that bladder training is less effective than surgery.
Explain to patients with post micturition dribble how to perform urethral milking.

Drug treatment
Offer drug treatment only to patients with **bothersome** lower urinary tract symptoms when conservative management options have been unsuccessful or are not appropriate.
Take into account comorbidities and current treatment when offering drug treatment for lower urinary tract symptoms.

Indication	Treatment	Review (assess symptoms and effect of the drugs on quality of life, and ask about any adverse effects)
Moderate to severe lower urinary tract symptoms	Offer an alpha blocker (alfuzosin, doxazosin, tamsulosin or terazosin)	At 4–6 weeks, then every 6–12 months
Overactive bladder	Offer an anticholinergic	At 4–6 weeks until stable, then every 6–12 months
	Mirabegron is recommended as an option for treating the symptoms of overactive bladder only for people in whom antimuscarinic drugs are contraindicated or clinically ineffective, or have unacceptable side effects. People currently receiving mirabegron that is not recommended for them above should be able to continue treatment until they and their clinician consider it appropriate to stop.	
Lower urinary tract symptoms and a prostate estimated to be larger than 30 g or PSA greater than 1.4 ng/ml, and high risk of progression	Offer a 5-alpha reductase inhibitor	At 3–6 months, then every 6–12 months
Bothersome moderate to severe lower urinary tract symptoms, and a prostate estimated to be larger than 30 g or PSA greater than 1.4 ng/ml	Consider an alpha blocker plus a 5-alpha reductase inhibitor	At 4–6 weeks, then every 6–12 months for the alpha blocker At 3–6 months, then every 6–12 months for the 5-alpha reductase inhibitor

Table (1): Treatment ladder for LUTS. (NICE guidelines)
Consider offering an anticholinergic as well as an alpha-blocker to patients who still have storage symptoms after treatment with an alpha-blocker alone.

Which anticholinergic to offer first?
The only available NICE guidance is on the treatment of UI (Urinary Incontinence) or OAB (Over active bladder) in females:
Offer one of the following choices first to female patients with OAB or mixed UI:
Oxybutynin (immediate release), or
Tolterodine (immediate release), or
Darifenacin (once daily preparation)
Do not offer oxybutynin to frail older patients.
If the first treatment for OAB or mixed UI is not effective or well-tolerated, offer another drug with the lowest acquisition cost.
Offer a transdermal OAB drug to patients unable to tolerate oral medication.
Mirabegron is recommended as an option for treating the symptoms of overactive bladder only for people in whom antimuscarinic drugs are contraindicated or clinically ineffective, or have unacceptable side effects.
Consider offering a late afternoon loop diuretic for nocturnal polyuria.
Consider offering oral desmopressin for nocturnal polyuria if other medical causes have been excluded and the patient has not benefited from other treatments. (Other medical causes include diabetes mellitus, diabetes insipidus, adrenal insufficiency, hypercalcaemia, liver failure, polyuric renal failure, chronic heart failure, obstructive apnoea, dependent oedema, pyelonephritis, chronic venous stasis, sickle cell anaemia, calcium channel blockers, diuretics, and selective serotonin reuptake inhibitors).
Measure serum sodium 3 days after the first dose.
If serum sodium is reduced to below the normal range, stop desmopressin treatment.
Do not offer phosphodiesterase-5-inhibitors solely for the purpose of treating lower urinary tract symptoms in men, except as part of a randomised controlled trial.
Do not offer homeopathy, phytotherapy or acupuncture.

Tadalafil for the treatment of symptoms associated with benign prostatic hyperplasia (terminated appraisal)
NICE is unable to make a recommendation about the use in the NHS of tadalafil for symptoms associated with benign prostatic hyperplasia.

If lower urinary tract symptoms do not respond to drug treatment
If lower urinary tract symptoms do not respond to drug treatment, discuss Active surveillance (reassurance and lifestyle advice without immediate treatment and with regular follow-up) or

Active intervention (conservative management or surgery).

Referral for specialist assessment
Refer patients for specialist assessment if they have:
Lower urinary tract symptoms complicated by recurrent or persistent urinary tract infection or
Retention or
Renal impairment you suspect is caused by lower urinary tract dysfunction or
Suspected urological cancer or
Stress urinary incontinence.
Offer to refer patients for specialist assessment if they have
Bothersome lower urinary tract symptoms that have not responded to conservative management or drug treatment.

Specialist assessment (Urologist) Important
Offer:
An assessment of general medical history to identify possible causes and comorbidities, including a review of all current medication (including herbal and over-the counter medication) that may be contributing to the problem.
A physical examination guided by symptoms and other medical conditions, an examination of the abdomen and external genitalia, and a digital rectal examination.
Flow-rate and post void residual volume measurement. (Note it is recommended in the specialist assessment but not the initial assessment which can be confusing)
Ask patients to complete a urinary frequency volume chart

When to offer further tests or procedures
Offer cystoscopy to patients with lower urinary tract symptoms having specialist assessment only when clinically indicated, for example if there is a history of any of the following:
Recurrent infection
Sterile pyuria
Haematuria
Profound symptoms
Pain

Offer imaging of the upper urinary tract to patients with lower urinary tract symptoms having specialist assessment only when clinically indicated, for example if there is a history of any of the following:
Chronic retention
Haematuria
Recurrent infection
Sterile pyuria
Profound symptoms
Pain

Consider offering multichannel cystometry if patients are considering surgery.
Offer pad tests only if the degree of urinary incontinence needs to be measured.

PSA testing
Offer patients information, advice and time to decide if they wish to have PSA testing if:
Their lower urinary tract symptoms are suggestive of bladder outlet obstruction secondary to benign prostate enlargement or
Their prostate feels abnormal on digital rectal examination or
They are concerned about prostate cancer (manage suspected prostate cancer in line with
the NICE pathways on prostate cancer and suspected cancer recognition and referral).

Acute retention
Immediately catheterise patients with acute retention.
Offer an alpha blocker to patients before removing the catheter.

Chronic urinary retention
Carry out a serum creatinine test and imaging of the upper urinary tract.
Impaired renal function or hydronephrosis
Catheterisation
Catheterise patients who have impaired renal function or hydronephrosis secondary to chronic urinary retention.
Consider offering intermittent or indwelling catheterisation before offering surgery (also see surgery in this pathway).
Consider offering intermittent self- or carer-administered urethral catheterisation before offering indwelling catheterisation.
If surgery is not suitable, continue or start long-term catheterisation (see long-term catheterisation and containment in this pathway).

Consider offering intermittent self- or carer-administered urethral catheterisation instead of surgery in patients who you suspect have markedly impaired bladder function. (usually patients with very large residuals > 2 litres)

Normal renal function and no hydronephrosis
If no bothersome LUTS
Catheterisation as above
Active surveillance
If not catheterising, provide active surveillance:
Post void residual volume measurement,
Upper tract imaging
Serum creatinine testing
If bothersome LUTS
Consider surgery without prior catheterisation
Consider offering surgery on the bladder outlet without prior catheterisation to patients who have chronic urinary retention and other bothersome lower urinary tract symptoms but no impairment of renal function or upper renal tract abnormality.

Surgery for voiding symptoms
Offer surgery only if voiding symptoms are severe or if drug treatment and conservative management options have been unsuccessful or are not appropriate. Discuss the alternatives to and outcomes from surgery.
Surgery for voiding lower urinary tract symptoms presumed secondary to benign prostate enlargement.

Prostate size	Type of surgery
All	Monopolar or bipolar TURP, monopolar TUVP or HoLEP. Perform HoLEP at a centre specialising in the technique, or with mentorship arrangements in place
Estimated to be smaller than 30 g	TUIP as an alternative to other types of surgery (TURP, monopolar TUVP or HoLEP)
Estimated to be larger than 80 g	TURP, TUVP or HoLEP, or open prostatectomy as an alternative. Perform HoLEP at a centre specialising in the technique, or with mentorship arrangements in place

Table (2): Surgical options for voiding symptoms.

If offering surgery to manage voiding lower urinary tract symptoms presumed secondary to benign prostate enlargement, offer botulinum toxin injection into the prostate only as part of a randomised controlled trial.
If offering surgery to manage voiding lower urinary tract symptoms presumed secondary to benign prostate enlargement, offer the following only as part of a randomised controlled trial that compares these techniques with TURP:
Laser vaporisation techniques
Bipolar TUVP
Monopolar or bipolar TUVRP.
Do not offer any of the following as an alternative to TURP, TUVP or HoLEP:
TUNA
TUMT
HIFU
TEAP
Laser coagulation.

Interventional procedures
Sacral nerve stimulation for idiopathic chronic non-obstructive urinary retention
Insertion of prostatic urethral lift implants to treat lower urinary tract symptoms secondary to benign prostatic hyperplasia.
Holmium laser prostatectomy.
Transurethral electrovaporisation of the prostate.
Laparoscopic prostatectomy for benign prostatic obstruction.
Prostate artery embolisation for benign prostatic hyperplasia.

Medical technologies
UroLift for treating lower urinary tract symptoms of benign prostatic hyperplasia
The clinical case for adopting the UroLift system for treating lower urinary tract symptoms of benign prostatic hyperplasia is supported by the evidence:
The UroLift system relieves lower urinary tract symptoms while:
Avoiding the risk to sexual function associated with transurethral resection of the prostate and holmium laser enucleation of the prostate.

Using the system Reduces the length of a person's stay in hospital. It can also be used in a day surgery unit.
The UroLift system should be considered as an alternative to current surgical procedures for use in a day case setting in patients with lower urinary tract symptoms of benign prostatic hyperplasia who are:

Aged 50 years and older and who have a:
Prostate of less than 100 ml
Without an obstructing middle lobe.

The TURis (transurethral resection in saline) system for transurethral resection of the prostate
The case for adopting the transurethral resection in saline (TURis) system for resection of the prostate is supported by the evidence. Using bipolar diathermy with TURis instead of a monopolar system
Avoids the risk of transurethral resection syndrome and:
Reduces the need for blood transfusion. It may also:
Reduce the length of hospital stay and hospital readmissions.

Surgery for storage symptoms
If offering surgery for storage symptoms, consider offering only to patients whose storage symptoms have not responded to conservative management and drug treatment. Discuss the alternatives of containment or surgery. Inform patients that effectiveness, side effects and long-term risks of surgery are uncertain.
Do not offer myectomy to manage detrusor over-activity.

Indication	Type of surgery
Detrusor over-activity	Consider offering: • Cystoplasty. Before offering, discuss serious complications (that is, bowel disturbance, metabolic acidosis, mucus production and/or mucus retention in the bladder, urinary tract infection and urinary retention). The man needs to be willing and able to self-catheterise. • Bladder wall injection with botulinum toxin. The man needs to be willing and able to self-catheterise. • Implanted sacral nerve stimulation.

Stress urinary incontinence	Consider offering: • implantation of an artificial sphincter. • intramural injectables, implanted adjustable compression devices and male slings only as part of a randomised controlled trial.
Intractable urinary tract symptoms if cystoplasty or sacral nerve stimulation are not clinically appropriate or are unacceptable to the man	Consider offering urinary diversion

Table (3): Surgical options for storage symptoms.
Interventional procedures

Percutaneous posterior tibial nerve stimulation for overactive bladder syndrome.
Laparoscopic augmentation cystoplasty (including clam cystoplasty).
Sacral nerve stimulation for urge incontinence and urgency-frequency.

Long-term catheterisation and containment
Consider offering long-term indwelling urethral catheterisation if medical management has failed and surgery is not appropriate, and the patient:
Is unable to manage intermittent self-catheterisation or
Has skin wounds, pressure ulcers or irritation that are being contaminated by urine or
Is distressed by bed and clothing changes.
Discuss the practicalities, benefits and risks of long-term indwelling catheterisation with the patient and, if appropriate, his carer.
Explain that indwelling catheters for urgency incontinence may not result in continence or the relief of recurrent infections.
Consider permanent use of containment products only after assessment and excluding other methods of management.

4.2. Prostate Cancer

Example scenario:
66-year-old man with PSA 5.3, How to assess?
History:
Full urological history (emphasis on LUTS)
Age
Racial origin
Family history
History of UTIs
Advanced disease suspected
Bone pain
Leg swelling
Anorexia
Weight loss
Coagulopathy
New-onset peripheral neurology
Examination
General urology examination
DRE
Further investigations
TRUS-guided prostate biopsy should be offered.
1% risk of severe bleeding or severe sepsis.
All patients experience some bleeding (rectal, haematuria, haematospermia) after procedure.
Treatment
Depends on grade/stage and patient comorbidities.
A man referred to clinic with high PSA how do you manage?

Do not automatically offer a Bx on the basis of serum PSA level alone.
If the clinical suspicion of prostate cancer is high, (high PSA and metastases) do not offer a prostate biopsy for histological confirmation, (only for clinical trial).
If Bx (-) discuss
There is still a risk that prostate cancer is present and
The risk is higher if:
HGPIN
ASAP
Abnormal DRE.

MRI for rebiopsy
Consider MRI (using T2- and diffusion-weighted imaging) for patients with a negative transrectal ultrasound 10–12 core biopsy.
Do not offer another biopsy if the multiparametric MRI is negative, unless any of the risk factors listed above are present.

Diagnostics
The PROGENSA PCA3 assay and the Prostate Health Index are not recommended for use in people who have had a negative or inconclusive trans-rectal ultrasound prostate biopsy.

Staging
Determine the provisional treatment intent (radical or non-radical) before decisions on imaging are made.
Do not routinely offer imaging to patients who are not candidates for radical treatment.
Offer isotope bone scans when hormonal therapy is being deferred through watchful waiting to asymptomatic patients who are at high risk of developing bone complications.
Consider multiparametric MRI, or CT if MRI is contraindicated, for patients with histologically proven prostate cancer if knowledge of the T or N stage could affect management.
Do not offer CT of the pelvis to patients with low- or intermediate-risk localised prostate cancer.
Do not routinely offer isotope bone scans to patients with low-risk localised prostate cancer.
Do not offer positron emission tomography imaging for prostate cancer in routine clinical practice.
Patients with localised or locally advanced prostate cancer:

Risk stratification for patients with localised prostate cancer

Level of risk	PSA (ng/ml)		Gleason score		Clinical stage
Low risk	<10	and	≤6	and	T1–T2a
Intermediate risk	10–20	or	7	or	T2b
High risk[1]	>20	or	8–10	or	≥T2c

Table (4): Risk stratification for men with localised prostate cancer (NICE guidelines)

Low-risk localised prostate cancer

Offer active surveillance as an option to men with low-risk localised prostate cancer for whom radical prostatectomy or radiotherapy is suitable.

Treatment options

Men with low-risk localised prostate cancer for whom radical prostatectomy or radical radiotherapy is suitable are also offered the option of active surveillance.

Rationale

Active surveillance can reduce overtreatment and increase capacity for rapid treatment of high-risk disease. It can also reduce the number of men unnecessarily having radical treatment and therefore experiencing adverse effects, and decrease the cost of treating and managing these adverse effects.

Intermediate-risk localised prostate cancer

Offer radical prostatectomy or radical radiotherapy to men with intermediate-risk localised prostate cancer.

Consider active surveillance for men with intermediate-risk localised prostate cancer who do not wish to have immediate radical prostatectomy or radiotherapy.

Do not offer bisphosphonates for the prevention of bone metastases in men with prostate cancer.

High-risk localised or locally advanced prostate cancer

Offer radical prostatectomy or radical radiotherapy to men with high-risk localised prostate cancer when there is a realistic prospect of long-term disease control.

Do not offer active surveillance to men with high-risk localised prostate cancer.

Do not offer bisphosphonates for the prevention of bone metastases in men with prostate cancer.

Protocol for active surveillance
Consider using the following protocol for men who have chosen active surveillance.

Timing	Tests
At enrolment in active surveillance	Multiparametric MRI if not previously performed[1]
Throughout active surveillance	Monitor PSA kinetics[2]
Year 1 of active surveillance	Every 3–4 months: measure PSA[3] Every 6–12 months: DRE[4] At 12 months: prostate rebiopsy[1]
Years 2–4 of active surveillance	Every 3–6 months: measure PSA[3] Every 6–12 months: DRE[4]
Year 5 and every year thereafter until active surveillance ends	Every 6 months: measure PSA[3] Every 12 months: DRE[4]

Table (5) Active surveillance protocol, NICE guidelines.
1 If there is concern about clinical or PSA changes at any time during active surveillance, reassess with multiparametric MRI and/or rebiopsy.
2 May include PSA doubling time and velocity.
3 May be carried out in primary care if there are agreed shared-care protocols and recall systems.
4 Should be performed by a healthcare professional with expertise and confidence in performing DRE

Information and support for men before starting radical treatment
Warn about alteration of sexual experience, possible loss of sexual function, and the potential loss of ejaculation and fertility. Offer sperm storage. Warn about effects of the treatment on urinary function.
Offer men experiencing troublesome LUTS before treatment a urological assessment.

There is a small increase in the risk of colorectal cancer after radical external beam radiotherapy for prostate cancer.

Radical treatment

Radical external beam radiotherapy

A minimum dose of 74 Gy to the prostate at no more than 2 Gy per fraction.

Androgen deprivation therapy

Offer men with intermediate- and high-risk localised prostate cancer a combination of radical radiotherapy and ADT, rather than radical radiotherapy or ADT alone.

Offer men with intermediate- and high-risk localised prostate cancer 6 months of ADT given before, during or after radical external beam radiotherapy.

Consider continuing ADT for up to 3 years for men with high-risk localised prostate cancer and discuss the benefits and risks of this option with them.

Brachytherapy

Consider high-dose rate brachytherapy in combination with external beam radiotherapy for men with intermediate- and high-risk localised prostate cancer.

Do not offer brachytherapy alone to men with high-risk localised prostate cancer.

Pelvic radiotherapy for locally advanced prostate cancer

Clinical oncologists should consider pelvic radiotherapy in men with locally advanced prostate cancer who have a greater than 15% risk of pelvic lymph node involvement and who are to receive neoadjuvant hormonal therapy and radical radiotherapy.

Pelvic lymph node involvement is estimated using the **Roach formula**:
% lymph node risk = 2/3 PSA + (10 × [Gleason score − 6]).

Interventions not recommended except in clinical trials:
High-intensity focused ultrasound or cryotherapy

Do not offer high-intensity focused ultrasound or cryotherapy to men with localised or locally advanced prostate cancer other than in the context of controlled clinical trials comparing their use with established interventions.

Postoperative radiotherapy
Do not offer immediate postoperative radiotherapy after radical prostatectomy, even to men with margin-positive disease, other than in the context of a clinical trial.

Hormonal therapy adjuvant to radical prostatectomy
Do not offer adjuvant hormonal therapy in addition to radical prostatectomy, even to men with margin-positive disease, other than in the context of a clinical trial.

Managing adverse effects of radical treatment

Sexual dysfunction
Early and ongoing access to specialist ED services.
Offer PDE5 inhibitors
If PDE5 inhibitors fail or contraindicated, offer vacuum devices, intraurethral inserts or penile
injections, or penile prostheses as an alternative.

Urinary incontinence
Access to specialist continence services
This may include coping strategies, along with pelvic floor muscle re-education, bladder retraining and pharmacotherapy.
Refer men with intractable stress incontinence to a specialist surgeon for consideration of an artificial urinary sphincter.
Do not offer injection of bulking agents into the distal urinary sphincter to treat stress incontinence.

Radiation-induced enteropathy
Offer care from a team of professionals with expertise in radiation-induced enteropathy (who may include oncologists, gastroenterologists, bowel surgeons, dietitians and specialist nurses).

Carry out full investigations, including flexible sigmoidoscopy, in men who have symptoms of radiation-induced enteropathy to exclude inflammatory bowel disease or malignancy of the large bowel and to ascertain the nature of the radiation injury.

Use caution when performing anterior wall rectal biopsy after brachytherapy because of the risk of fistulation.

Managing relapse after radical treatment

Do not offer biopsy of the prostatic bed to men with prostate cancer who have had a radical prostatectomy.

Offer biopsy of the prostate after radiotherapy only to men with prostate cancer who are being considered for local salvage therapy in the context of a clinical trial.

For men with evidence of biochemical relapse following radical treatment and who are considering radical salvage therapy:

do not offer routine MRI scanning prior to salvage radiotherapy in men with prostate cancer

offer an isotope bone scan if symptoms or PSA trends are suggestive of metastases.

Biochemical relapse (a rising PSA) alone should not necessarily prompt an immediate change in treatment.

Biochemical relapse should trigger an estimate of PSA doubling time, based on a minimum of 3 measurements over at least a 6-month period.

Offer men with biochemical relapse after radical prostatectomy, with no known metastases, radical radiotherapy to the prostatic bed.

Men with biochemical relapse should be considered for entry to appropriate clinical trials.

Do not routinely offer hormonal therapy to men with prostate cancer who have a biochemical relapse unless they have:

Symptomatic local disease progression or

Any proven metastases or

A PSA doubling time of less than 3 months.

Hormone therapy

Consider intermittent therapy for men having long-term ADT (not in the adjuvant setting), and discuss:

the limited evidence for reduction in side effects from intermittent therapy and

the effect of intermittent therapy on progression of prostate cancer.

Based on the schedules in use in clinical trials,

treatment is stopped when the PSA is < 4 ng/mL after 6 to 7 months of treatment.

Treatment is resumed when the PSA is > 10-20 ng/mL
For men who are having intermittent ADT:
measure PSA every 3 months and
restart ADT if PSA is 10 ng/ml or above, or if there is symptomatic progression.

Types of anti-androgens (Important)
Non-steroidal anti-androgens (e.g. bicalutamide, flutamide) They block androgen at receptor level
Steroidal anti-androgens (e.g. cyproterone acetate) They down-regulate LHRH secretion by having additional progesterogenic activity and also block androgen at receptor level

How does Oestrogen work?
It down-regulates LHRH secretion and inactivates androgen and suppresses Leydig cells.

Managing adverse effects of hormone therapy

Hot flushes
Offer medroxyprogesterone[1] (20 mg per day), initially for 10 weeks, to manage troublesome hot flushes.
Consider cyproterone acetate (50 mg twice a day for 4 weeks) if medroxyprogesterone is not
effective or not tolerated.
Tell men that there is no good-quality evidence for the use of complementary therapies to treat troublesome hot flushes.

Sexual dysfunction
Access to specialist erectile dysfunction services.
Psychosexual counselling.
Offer PDE5 inhibitors
If PDE5 inhibitors fail to restore erectile function or are contraindicated, offer a choice of:
intraurethral inserts
penile injections
penile prostheses
vacuum devices.

Osteoporosis
Do not routinely offer bisphosphonates to prevent osteoporosis in men with prostate cancer having ADT.
Consider assessing fracture risk in men with prostate cancer who are having ADT, in line with fragility fracture risk assessment in the NICE pathway on osteoporosis.

Offer bisphosphonates to men who are having ADT and have osteoporosis.

Consider denosumab for men who are having ADT and have osteoporosis if bisphosphonates are contraindicated or not tolerated.

Gynaecomastia

For men starting long-term (longer than 6 months) bicalutamide monotherapy, offer
prophylactic radiotherapy to both breast buds within the first month of treatment. Choose a single fraction of 8 Gy using orthovoltage or electron beam radiotherapy.

If radiotherapy is unsuccessful in preventing gynaecomastia, weekly tamoxifen[2] should be considered.

Fatigue

Offer men who are starting or having ADT supervised resistance and aerobic exercise at least twice a week for 12 weeks to reduce fatigue and improve quality of life.

Follow-up

Check PSA levels for all men with prostate cancer who are having radical treatment at the earliest 6 weeks following treatment, at least every 6 months for the first 2 years and then at least once a year thereafter.

Do not routinely offer DRE to men with localised prostate cancer while the PSA remains at baseline levels.

After at least 2 years, offer follow-up outside hospital (for example, in primary care) by telephone or secure electronic communications to men with a stable PSA who have had no significant treatment complications, unless they are taking part in a clinical trial that requires formal clinic-based follow-up.

Men who have chosen a watchful waiting regimen

Men with prostate cancer who have chosen a watchful waiting regimen with no curative intent should normally be followed up in primary care in accordance with protocols agreed by the local urological cancer MDT and the relevant primary care organisation(s). Their PSA should be measured at least once a year.

Information and support

Access to specialist urology and palliative care teams

Offer a regular assessment of needs to men with metastatic prostate cancer.

Palliative care

Integrate palliative interventions at any stage into coordinated care, and facilitate any transitions between care settings as smoothly as possible.

Discuss personal preferences for palliative care as early as possible with men with metastatic prostate cancer, their partners and carers. Tailor treatment/care plans accordingly and identify the preferred place of care.

Ensure that palliative care is available when needed and is not limited to the end of life. It should not be restricted to being associated with hospice care.

Treatment

Offer bilateral orchidectomy to all men with metastatic prostate cancer as an alternative to continuous LHRH agonist therapy.

Do not offer combined androgen blockage as a first-line treatment for men with metastatic prostate cancer.

For men with metastatic prostate cancer who are willing to accept the adverse impact on overall survival and gynaecomastia in the hope of retaining sexual function, offer anti-androgen monotherapy with bicalutamide (150 mg)[1].

Begin ADT and stop bicalutamide treatment in men with metastatic prostate cancer who are taking bicalutamide monotherapy and who do not maintain satisfactory sexual function.

Denosumab for men with bone metastases

Denosumab is not recommended for preventing skeletal-related events in adults with bone metastases from prostate cancer.

Adults with bone metastases from solid tumours currently receiving denosumab for the prevention of skeletal-related events that is not recommended according to the criteria above should be able to continue treatment until they and their clinician consider it appropriate to stop.

Corticosteroids

Offer a corticosteroid such as dexamethasone (0.5 mg daily) as third-line hormonal therapy after ADT and anti-androgen therapy to men with hormone-relapsed prostate cancer.

Bone metastases

Spinal MRI

Do not routinely offer spinal MRI to all men with hormone-relapsed prostate cancer and known bone metastases.

Offer spinal MRI to men with hormone-relapsed prostate cancer shown to have extensive metastases in the spine (for example, on a bone scan) if they develop any spinal-related symptoms.

Bone-targeted therapies
Bisphosphonates
Do not offer bisphosphonates to prevent or reduce the complications of bone metastases in men with hormone-relapsed metastatic prostate cancer.

Bisphosphonates for pain relief may be considered for men with hormone-relapsed prostate cancer when other treatments (including analgesics and palliative radiotherapy) have failed. Choose the oral or intravenous route of administration according to convenience, tolerability and cost.

Strontium-89
Strontium-89 should be considered for men with hormone-relapsed prostate cancer and painful bone metastases, especially those men who are unlikely to receive myelosuppressive chemotherapy.

Radium-223 dichloride
Radium-223 dichloride is recommended as an option for treating adults with hormone-relapsed prostate cancer, symptomatic bone metastases and no known visceral metastases, only if:

they have had treatment with docetaxel, and

the company provides radium-223 dichloride with the discount agreed in the patient access scheme.

Denosumab
Denosumab is not recommended for preventing skeletal-related events in adults with bone metastases from prostate cancer.

Obstructive uropathy
Offer decompression of the upper urinary tract by percutaneous nephrostomy or by insertion of a double J stent to men with obstructive uropathy secondary to hormone-relapsed prostate cancer.

The option of no intervention should also be discussed with men with obstructive uropathy secondary to hormone-relapsed prostate cancer and remains a choice for some.

Treatment options before chemotherapy
Enzalutamide
Enzalutamide is recommended, within its marketing authorisation, as an option for treating metastatic hormone-relapsed prostate cancer:

in people who have no or mild symptoms after androgen deprivation therapy has failed, and before chemotherapy is indicated

when the company provides it with the discount agreed in the patient access scheme.

Chemotherapy
Docetaxel
Docetaxel is recommended, within its licensed indications, as a treatment option for men with hormone-refractory metastatic prostate cancer only if their Karnofsky performance-status score is 60% or more.
It is recommended that treatment with docetaxel should be stopped:
at the completion of planned treatment of up to 10 cycles or
if severe adverse events occur or
in the presence of progression of disease as evidenced by clinical or laboratory criteria, or by imaging studies.
Repeat cycles of treatment with docetaxel are not recommended if the disease recurs after completion of the planned course of chemotherapy.

Treatment options after chemotherapy
Enzalutamide
Enzalutamide is a rationally designed oral AR inhibitor that inhibits multiple steps in the Androgen Receptor (AR) signaling pathway. The mechanism of action for enzalutamide is threefold. It is a potent, competitive binder of androgens at the level of the AR. It prevents the translocation of the AR from the cytoplasm to the nucleus. Within the nucleus, it inhibits AR binding to chromosomal DNA, which prevents further transcription of tumor genes.
Enzalutamide is recommended within its marketing authorisation as an option for treating metastatic hormone relapsed prostate cancer in adults whose disease has progressed **during or after** docetaxel-containing chemotherapy, only if the manufacturer provides enzalutamide with the discount agreed in the patient access scheme.

Abiraterone
Mechanism of action: Inhibition of **CYP17** activity which is required for androgen biosynthesis thus decreases circulating levels of androgens such as DHEA, testosterone, and dihydrotestosterone (DHT).
Abiraterone in combination with prednisone or prednisolone is recommended as an option for the treatment of castration-resistant **metastatic** prostate cancer in adults, only if:
Their disease has progressed **on or after** one docetaxel-containing chemotherapy regimen and
The manufacturer provides abiraterone with the discount agreed in the patient access scheme.

Cabazitaxel

Cabazitaxel in combination with prednisone or prednisolone is not recommended for the treatment of hormone-refractory metastatic prostate cancer previously treated with a docetaxel-containing regimen.

4.3. Bladder Cancer

Bladder Cancer Nice guidelines
Non-muscle-invasive bladder cancer
Risk classification in non-muscle-invasive bladder cancer

There is no widely accepted classification of risk in non-muscle-invasive bladder cancer. To make clear recommendations for management, the Guideline Development Group developed the consensus classification in the table below, based on the evidence reviewed and clinical opinion.

Low risk	Urothelial cancer with any of: • solitary pTaG1 with a diameter of less than 3 cm • solitary pTaG2 (low grade) with a diameter of less than 3 cm • any papillary urothelial neoplasm of low malignant potential
Intermediate risk	Urothelial cancer that is not low risk or high risk, including: • solitary pTaG1 with a diameter of more than 3 cm • multifocal pTaG1 • solitary pTaG2 (low grade) with a diameter of more than 3 cm • multifocal pTaG2 (low grade)

	- pTaG2 (high grade) - any pTaG2 (grade not further specified) - any low-risk non-muscle-invasive bladder cancer recurring within 12 months of last tumour occurrence
High risk	Urothelial cancer with any of: - pTaG3 - pT1G2 - pT1G3 - pTis (Cis) - aggressive variants of urothelial carcinoma, for example micropapillary or nested variants

Table (6): Risk categories in non-muscle-invasive bladder cancer

Prognostic markers and risk classification

Ensure that for people with non-muscle-invasive bladder cancer all of the following are recorded and used to guide discussions, both within multidisciplinary team meetings and with the person, about prognosis and treatment options:

recurrence history

size and number of cancers

histological type, grade, stage and presence (or absence) of flat urothelium, detrusor muscle (muscularis propria), and carcinoma in situ

the risk category of the person's cancer

predicted risk of recurrence and progression, estimated using a risk prediction tool.

Low-risk non-muscle-invasive bladder cancer

For the treatment of low-risk non-muscle-invasive bladder cancer, Offer white-light-guided TURBT with one of photodynamic diagnosis, narrow-band imaging, cytology or a urinary biomarker test (such as UroVysion using fluorescence in-situ hybridization [FISH], ImmunoCyt or a nuclear matrix protein 22 [NMP22] test) to people with suspected bladder cancer. This should be carried out or supervised by a urologist experienced in TURBT.

Obtain detrusor muscle during TURBT.

Do not take random biopsies of normal-looking urothelium during TURBT unless there is a specific clinical indication (for example, investigation of positive cytology not otherwise explained).

Record the size and number of tumours during TURBT.

Offer people with suspected bladder cancer a single dose of intravesical mitomycin C given at the same time as the first TURBT.

Staging

Consider further TURBT within 6 weeks if the first specimen does not include detrusor muscle.

Intermediate-risk non-muscle-invasive bladder cancer

Offer people with newly diagnosed intermediate-risk non-muscle-invasive bladder cancer a course of at least 6 doses of intravesical mitomycin C.

If intermediate-risk non-muscle-invasive bladder cancer recurs after a course of intravesical mitomycin C, refer the person's care to a specialist urology multidisciplinary team.

High-risk non-muscle-invasive bladder cancer

If the first TURBT shows high-risk non-muscle-invasive bladder cancer, offer another TURBT as soon as possible and no later than 6 weeks after the first resection.

Offer the choice of intravesical BCG (Bacille Calmette-Guérin) or radical cystectomy to people with high-risk non-muscle-invasive bladder cancer, and base the choice on a full discussion with the person, the clinical nurse specialist and a urologist who performs both intravesical BCG and radical cystectomy. **Include in your discussion**:

The type, stage and grade of the cancer, the presence of carcinoma in situ, the presence of variant pathology, prostatic urethral or bladder neck status and the number of tumours

Risk of progression to muscle invasion, metastases and death

Risk of understaging

Benefits of both treatments, including survival rates and the likelihood of further treatment

Risks of both treatments

Factors that affect outcomes (for example, comorbidities and life expectancy)

Impact on quality of life, body image, and sexual and urinary function.

Intravesical BCG

Offer induction and maintenance intravesical BCG to people having treatment with intravesical BCG.

If induction BCG fails (because it is not tolerated, or bladder cancer persists or recurs after treatment with BCG), refer the person's care to a specialist urology multidisciplinary team.

For people in whom induction BCG has failed, the specialist urology multidisciplinary team should assess the suitability of radical cystectomy, or further intravesical therapy if radical cystectomy is unsuitable or declined by the person, or if the bladder cancer that recurs is intermediate- or low-risk.

Recurrent non-muscle--invasive bladder cancer
Consider fulguration without biopsy for people with recurrent non-muscle-invasive bladder cancer if they have all of the following:
no previous bladder cancer that was intermediate- or high-risk
a disease-free interval of at least 6 months
solitary papillary recurrence
a tumour diameter of 3 mm or less.

Managing side effects of treatment
Do not offer primary prophylaxis to prevent BCG-related bladder toxicity except as part of a clinical trial.
Seek advice from a specialist urology multidisciplinary team if symptoms of bladder toxicity after BCG cannot be controlled with antispasmodics or non-opiate analgesia and other causes have been excluded by cystoscopy.

Follow-up after treatment for non-muscle-invasive bladder cancer
Refer people urgently to urological services if they have haematuria or other urinary symptoms and a history of non-muscle-invasive bladder cancer.

Low-risk non-muscle-invasive bladder cancer
Offer people with low-risk non-muscle-invasive bladder cancer cystoscopic follow-up 3 months and 12 months after diagnosis.
Do not use urinary biomarkers or cytology in addition to cystoscopy for follow-up after treatment for low-risk bladder cancer.
Discharge to primary care people who have had low-risk non-muscle-invasive bladder cancer and who have no recurrence of the bladder cancer within 12 months.
Do not offer routine urinary cytology or prolonged cystoscopic follow-up after 12 months for people with low-risk non-muscle-invasive bladder cancer.

Intermediate-risk non-muscle-invasive bladder cancer
Offer people with intermediate-risk non-muscle-invasive bladder cancer cystoscopic follow-up at 3, 9 and 18 months, and once a year thereafter.
Consider discharging people who have had intermediate-risk non-muscle-invasive bladder cancer to primary care after 5 years of disease-free follow-up.

High-risk non-muscle-invasive bladder cancer
Offer people with high-risk non-muscle-invasive bladder cancer cystoscopic follow-up:
every 3 months for the first 2 years **then**
every 6 months for the next 2 years **then**
once a year thereafter.

Diagnosis and staging
Diagnosing and staging bladder cancer
Diagnosis
Do not substitute urinary biomarkers for cystoscopy to investigate suspected bladder cancer or for follow-up after treatment for bladder cancer, except in the context of a clinical research study.

Consider CT or MRI staging before transurethral resection of bladder tumour (TURBT) **if muscle-invasive bladder cancer is suspected at cystoscopy.**

Offer white-light-guided TURBT with one of photodynamic diagnosis, narrow-band imaging, cytology or a urinary biomarker test (such as UroVysion using fluorescence in-situ hybridization [FISH], ImmunoCyt or a nuclear matrix protein 22 [NMP22] test) to people with suspected bladder cancer. This should be carried out or supervised by a urologist experienced in TURBT.

Obtain detrusor muscle during TURBT.

Do not take random biopsies of normal-looking urothelium during TURBT unless there is a specific clinical indication (for example, investigation of positive cytology not otherwise explained).

Record the size and number of tumours during TURBT.

Offer people with suspected bladder cancer a single dose of intravesical mitomycin C given at the same time as the first TURBT.

Staging
Consider further TURBT within 6 weeks if the first specimen does not include detrusor muscle.

Offer CT or MRI staging to people diagnosed with muscle-invasive bladder cancer or high-risk non-muscle-invasive bladder cancer that is being assessed for radical treatment.

Consider CT urography, carried out with other planned CT imaging if possible, to detect upper tract involvement in people with new or recurrent high-risk non-muscle-invasive or muscle-invasive bladder cancer.

Consider CT of the thorax, carried out with other planned CT imaging if possible, to detect thoracic malignancy in people with muscle-invasive bladder cancer.

Consider fluorodeoxyglucose positron emission tomography (FDG PET)-CT for people with muscle-invasive bladder cancer or high-risk non-muscle-invasive bladder cancer before radical treatment if there are indeterminate findings on CT or MRI, or a high risk of metastatic disease (for example, T3b disease).

Muscle-invasive bladder cancer

TNM Classification:

T- Primary Tumour
T2 Tumour invades muscle
T2a Tumour invades superficial muscle (inner half)
T2b Tumour invades deep muscle (outer half)
T3 Tumour invades perivesical tissue:
T3a Microscopically
T3b Macroscopically (extravesical mass)
T4 Tumour invades any of the following: prostate stroma, seminal vesicles, uterus, vagina, pelvic wall, abdominal wall.
T4a Tumour invades prostate stroma, seminal vesicles, uterus, or vagina
T4b Tumour invades pelvic wall or abdominal wall
N- Regional Lymph Nodes
Nx Regional lymph nodes cannot be assessed
N0 no regional lymph nodes metastases
N1 Metastasis in a single lymph node in the true pelvis (hypogastric, obturator, external iliac, or presacral)

N2 Metastasis in multiple lymph nodes in the true pelvis (hypogastric, obturator, external iliac, or presacral)
N3 Metastasis in common iliac lymph nodes
M- Distant metastasis
M0 No distant metastasis
M1 Distant metastasis

Treating muscle-invasive bladder cancer
Ensure that a specialist urology multidisciplinary team reviews all cases of muscle-invasive bladder cancer, including adenocarcinoma, squamous cell carcinoma and neuroendocrine carcinoma, and that the review includes histopathology, imaging and discussion of treatment options.

Neoadjuvant chemotherapy for newly diagnosed muscle-invasive urothelial bladder cancer
Offer neoadjuvant chemotherapy using a cisplatin combination regimen before radical cystectomy or radical radiotherapy to people with newly diagnosed muscle-invasive urothelial bladder cancer for whom cisplatin-based chemotherapy is suitable. Ensure that they have an opportunity to discuss the risks and benefits with an oncologist who TLtreats bladder cancer.

Radical therapy for muscle-invasive urothelial bladder cancer
Offer a choice of radical cystectomy or radiotherapy with a radiosensitiser to people with muscle-invasive urothelial bladder cancer for whom radical therapy is suitable. Ensure that the choice is based on a full discussion between the person and a urologist who performs radical cystectomy, a clinical oncologist and a clinical nurse specialist. Include in the discussion:
the prognosis with or without treatment
the limited evidence about whether surgery or radiotherapy with a radiosensitiser is the most effective cancer treatment
the benefits and risks of surgery and radiotherapy with a radiosensitiser, including the impact on sexual and bowel function and the risk of death as a result of the treatment.

Factors that favour cystectomy:
Presence of CIS
Upper tract obstruction

Presence of inflammatory bowel disease
Presence of severe irritative urinary symptoms
Previous extensive abdominal surgery
Previous pelvic radiotherapy
Young patient.

Radical cystectomy
Offer people who have chosen radical cystectomy a urinary stoma, or a continent urinary diversion (bladder substitution or a catheterisable reservoir) if there are no strong contraindications to continent urinary diversion such as cognitive impairment, impaired renal function or significant bowel disease.
Members of the specialist urology multidisciplinary team (including the bladder cancer specialist urological surgeon, stoma care nurse and clinical nurse specialist) should discuss with the person whether to have a urinary stoma or continent urinary diversion, and provide opportunities for the person to talk with people who have had these procedures.
Offer people with bladder cancer and, if they wish, their partners, families or carers, opportunities to have discussions with a stoma care nurse before and after radical cystectomy as needed.

Adjuvant chemotherapy after radical cystectomy for muscle-invasive or lymph-node-positive urothelial bladder cancer
Consider adjuvant cisplatin combination chemotherapy after radical cystectomy for people with a diagnosis of muscle-invasive or lymph-node-positive urothelial bladder cancer for whom neoadjuvant chemotherapy was not suitable (because muscle invasion was not shown on biopsies before cystectomy). Ensure that the person has an opportunity to discuss the risks and benefits with an oncologist who treats bladder cancer.

Radical radiotherapy
Use a radiosensitiser (such as mitomycin in combination with fluorouracil [5-FU][1] or carbogen in combination with nicotinamide[2]) when giving radical radiotherapy (for example, 64 Gy in 32 fractions over 6.5 weeks or 55 Gy in 20 fractions over 4 weeks) for muscle-invasive urothelial bladder cancer.

Managing side effects of treatment
Seek advice from a specialist urology multidisciplinary team if symptoms of bladder toxicity after radiotherapy cannot be controlled with

antispasmodics or non-opiate analgesia and other causes have been excluded by cystoscopy.

Follow-up after treatment for muscle-invasive bladder cancer

Offer follow-up after radical cystectomy or radical radiotherapy.

After radical cystectomy consider using a follow-up protocol that consists of:

monitoring of the upper tracts for hydronephrosis, stones and cancer using imaging and glomerular filtration rate (GFR) estimation at least annually **and**

monitoring for local and distant recurrence using CT of the abdomen, pelvis and chest, carried out together with other planned CT imaging if possible, 6, 12 and 24 months after radical cystectomy **and**

monitoring for metabolic acidosis and B12 and folate deficiency at least annually **and**

for men with a defunctioned urethra, urethral washing for cytology and/or urethroscopy annually for 5 years to detect urethral recurrence.

After radical radiotherapy consider using a follow-up protocol that includes all of the following:

rigid cystoscopy 3 months after radiotherapy has been completed, followed by either rigid or flexible cystoscopy:

every 3 months for the first 2 years **then**

every 6 months for the next 2 years **then**

every year thereafter, according to clinical judgement and the person's preference

upper-tract imaging every year for 5 years

monitoring for local and distant recurrence using CT of the abdomen, pelvis and chest, carried out with other planned CT imaging if possible, 6, 12 and 24 months after radical radiotherapy has finished.

Locally advanced or metastatic muscle-invasive bladder cancer

Managing locally advanced or metastatic muscle-invasive bladder cancer

First-line chemotherapy

Discuss the role of first-line chemotherapy with people who have locally advanced or metastatic bladder cancer. Include in your discussion:

prognosis of their cancer **and**

advantages and disadvantages of the treatment options, including best supportive care.

Offer a cisplatin-based chemotherapy regimen (such as cisplatin in combination with gemcitabine, or accelerated [high-dose] methotrexate, vinblastine, doxorubicin and cisplatin [MVAC] in combination with granulocyte-colony stimulating factor [G-CSF]) to people with locally advanced or metastatic urothelial bladder cancer who are otherwise physically fit (have an Eastern Cooperative Oncology Group [ECOG] performance status of 0 or 1) and have adequate renal function (typically defined as a glomerular filtration rate [GFR] of 60 ml/min/1.73 m² or more).

Offer carboplatin in combination with gemcitabine[3] to people with locally advanced or metastatic urothelial bladder cancer with an ECOG performance status of 0–2 if a cisplatin-based chemotherapy regimen is unsuitable, for example, because of ECOG performance status, inadequate renal function (typically defined as a GFR of less than 60 ml/min/1.73 m²) or comorbidity. Assess and discuss the risks and benefits with the person.

For people having first-line chemotherapy for locally advanced or metastatic bladder cancer:

carry out regular clinical and radiological monitoring **and**

actively manage symptoms of disease and treatment-related toxicity **and**

stop first-line chemotherapy if there is excessive toxicity or disease progression.

Second-line chemotherapy

Discuss second-line chemotherapy with people who have locally advanced or metastatic bladder cancer. Include in your discussion:

the prognosis of their cancer

advantages and disadvantages of treatment options, including best supportive care.

Consider second-line chemotherapy with gemcitabine in combination with cisplatin, or accelerated (high-dose) MVAC in combination with G-CSF for people with incurable locally advanced or metastatic urothelial bladder cancer whose condition has progressed after first-line chemotherapy if:

their renal function is adequate (typically defined as a GFR of 60 ml/min/1.73 m² or more) **and**

they are otherwise physically fit (have an ECOG performance status of 0 or 1).

Consider second-line chemotherapy with carboplatin in combination with paclitaxel[3] or gemcitabine in combination with paclitaxel[4] for people with incurable locally advanced or metastatic urothelial bladder cancer for whom cisplatin-based chemotherapy is not suitable, or who choose not to have it.

For recommendations on vinflunine as second-line chemotherapy for people with incurable locally advanced or metastatic urothelial bladder cancer, see NICE's technology appraisal guidance on vinflunine for the treatment of advanced or metastatic transitional cell carcinoma of the urothelial tract.

For people having second-line chemotherapy for locally advanced or metastatic bladder cancer:

carry out regular clinical and radiological monitoring **and**

actively manage symptoms of disease and treatment-related toxicity **and**

stop second-line chemotherapy if there is excessive toxicity or disease progression.

Managing symptoms of locally advanced or metastatic bladder cancer
Bladder symptoms

Offer palliative hypofractionated radiotherapy to people with symptoms of haematuria, dysuria, urinary frequency or nocturia caused by advanced bladder cancer that is unsuitable for potentially curative treatment.

Loin pain and symptoms of renal failure

Discuss treatment options with people who have locally advanced or metastatic bladder cancer with ureteric obstruction. Include in your discussion:

prognosis of their cancer **and**

advantages and disadvantages of the treatment options, including best supportive care.

Consider percutaneous nephrostomy or retrograde stenting (if technically feasible) for people with locally advanced or metastatic bladder cancer and ureteric obstruction who need treatment to relieve pain, treat acute kidney injury or improve renal function before further treatment.

If facilities for percutaneous nephrostomy or retrograde stenting are not available at the local hospital, or if these procedures are unsuccessful, discuss the options with a specialist urology multidisciplinary team for people with bladder cancer and ureteric obstruction.

Intractable bleeding

Evaluate the cause of intractable bleeding with the local urology team.
Consider hypofractionated radiotherapy or embolisation for people with intractable bleeding caused by incurable bladder cancer.

If a person has intractable bleeding caused by bladder cancer and radiotherapy or embolisation are not suitable treatments, discuss further management with a specialist urology multidisciplinary team.

Pelvic pain

Evaluate the cause of pelvic pain with the local urology team.

Consider, in addition to best supportive care, 1 or more of the following to treat **pelvic pain caused by incurable bladder cancer:**

hypofractionated radiotherapy if the person has not had pelvic radiotherapy

nerve block

palliative chemotherapy.

Specialist palliative care for people with incurable bladder cancer

A member of the treating team should offer people with incurable bladder cancer a sensitive explanation that their disease cannot be cured and refer them to the urology multidisciplinary team.

Tell the primary care team that the person has been given a diagnosis of incurable bladder cancer within 24 hours of telling the person.

A member of the urology multidisciplinary team should discuss the prognosis and management options with people with incurable bladder cancer.

Discuss palliative care services with people with incurable bladder cancer and, if needed and they agree, refer them to a specialist palliative care team.

Offer people with symptomatic incurable bladder cancer access to a urological team with the full range of options for managing symptoms.

4.4. Testicular Cancer

26-year-old referred with right sided testicular mass how to assess.
History

- Duration of symptoms
- Painful or painless mass
- Change in size of mass
- Any previous history of surgery on the genitalia
- Sexual history: recent sexual contact or penile discharge
- Associate urinary symptoms
- Trauma
- Differential diagnosis: hydrocele, varicocele, sebaceous cyst, hernia, epididymal cyst, scrotal stone, sperm granuloma)

Previous relevant history and risk factors (Important)
History of cryptorchidism (on either side)
Increases the risk of testicular cancer in the undescended testicle by 4-13 times.
Family history of testicular cancer
Especially in fathers and brothers increases the risk by 6 and 8 times.
Racial origin

Three times more common in Caucasians and in Northern Europe, with the highest incidence in Scandinavia. (11/100000) In UK (7/100000)

Maternal oestrogen exposure
Fetal exposure to diethylstilboestrol increases the risk by 2.8-5.3 %

History of subfertility
Increases the risk by 1.6 times.

Contralateral history of testicular tumour
5-10% risk of cancer in the remaining testicle

HIV
Increased risk of seminoma

Physical examination
Palpation of supraclavicular nodes
Chest examination
Abdominal examination to palpate for retroperitoneal nodal mass
Check for inguinal scars from childhood orchidopexy
Examine testicle for the mass, size, painful painless, examine contralateral testicle.

Differential diagnosis of scrotal lump: (Important)
Inguinal hernia
Hydrocele
Epididymal cyst
Varicocele
Sebaceous cyst
Tuberculous epididymo-orchitis
Gumma of the testis
Carcinoma of scrotal skin

Investigations if suspicious
Urgent ultrasound scan (has almost 100% sensitivity for testicular tumour detection)
Walk the patient to the radiology department

If USS confirms tumour any other investigations

Tumour markers
AFP (half-life 5 days)
bHCG (half-life 36 hours)
LDH (half-life 3 days)

Chest xray
Note: Presence of widespread testicular metastases on chest X-ray is an **oncological emergency, and the patient must be referred urgently to an**

oncologist. Immediate chemotherapy may be necessary prior to radical inguinal orchidectomy in these cases).

Do all patients have raised tumour markers?
51% of all testicular tumours will have raised tumour markers.
Seminomas
5-10% of pure seminomas will have a raised bhCG
Pure seminomas do not secrete AFP
10% have raised LDH levels
NSGCT
50-70% of NSGCT have raised AFP
40% of NSGCT have raised BhCG
Other
100% of choriocarcinomas have raised BhCG
40-60% of embryonal carcinoma have raised BhCG
What is the role of tumour markers?
Diagnostic
Prognostic
Post orchidectomy measurement is useful in assessing the likelihood of retroperitoneal and metastatic disease.
What is the significance of measuring LDH?
Determines tumour burden
Surrogate marker for tumour volume and cell necrosis
Helpful for seminomas as a measure of tumour response
What else can raise tumour markers?
BhCG can be raised in the following cancers
Liver
Pancreatic
Stomach
Lung
Breast
Kidney
Bladder
and in
Marijuana smokers
Hypogonadotrophic patients raised LH may cross-react with some radioimmunoassay techniques for BhCG
AFP can be raised in the following cancers

Liver
Pancreas
Stomach
Lung
Benign liver dysfunction

Post-operative imaging?
If GCT is confirmed
Staging CT Abdo and pelvis is performed
NSGCT
Chest CT is undertaken
Chest CT is not mandatory of sage I seminoma according to EAU guidelines

Roles of MRI and PET
MRI to assess retroperitoneal nodes in patients with contrast allergy
PET to assess residual retroperiotneal mass after chemotherapy can be safely watched or whether it requires active treatment.

Management of this patient
Urgent radical inguinal orchidectomy (generally within 1 week)
Assess whether contralateral testicular biopsy is required

How would you perform a radical inguinal orchidectomy?
An inguinal incision.
Prior to manipulation of the testis the cord is isolated and clamped to allow control of the draining lymphatics to minimize tumour spill towards the retroperitoneal nodes.
The tumour-bearing testicle and cord are mobilised to the deep inguinal ring.
The cord is transected and secured with one heavy tie (0 or 1 vicryl) and an additional transfixing suture. Some authors suggest that a prolene suture should be used at the cut end of the cord to act as a marker for possible future nodal dissection.

Complications
Bleeding
Infection
loss of sensation on the inner thigh and ipsilateral scrotal wall
chronic groin pain (damage to ilioinguinal nerve)
Anything else you offer patient prior to orchidectomy?
Sperm banking
Insertion of testicular prosthesis

EAU recommends Cryopreservation of sperm prior to orchidectomy

Banking is advisable if
History of sub-fertility
Small contralateral testicle
Fertility is an issue for the patient

Prosthesis
Should be offered at the same sitting
Caution in patients likely to need early post-operative chemotherapy (Pulmonary metastases, markedly raised markers) because prosthesis related infection (0.6-2%) may delay this.

How patients bank sperm?
Attend a designated fertility clinic
Provide three semen samples with a 2-3-day period of abstinence.
Brief assessment of sperm quality is undertaken microscopically
Sample is then frozen in liquid nitrogen at −196C.
Patient should be made aware of the following
quality of sperm is not guaranteed when thawed.
Illness prior to banking sperm may affect the quality of the sperm
Banking can still be done in the first week or so following initiation of chemotherapy.
Some evidence that quality of sperm in men with GCT is poor compared with matched healthy males, assisted techniques might be required.
Maximum storage period is 10 years
All men should be screened for HIV and for hepatitis B and C. Men with HIV can bank sperm in separate storage vessels.
The cost for the first year is met by the NHS, thereafter the patient pays 200£ per year of storage.
Patient might need to travel some distance to bank sperm.

Complications of testicular prosthesis
Extrusion from scrotum (3-8%)
Scrotal contraction and migration (3-5%)
Chronic pain (1-3%)
Haematoma (0.3-3%)
Infection (0.6-2%)

Who should have contralateral testicular biopsy?
To identify ITGCN (5-9%) risk in patients with testicular cancer.
Men under the age of 40
Testis volume < 12 ml
History of undescended testis and subfertility.

What pathological info you need?
Histological type of tumour (germ-cell tumour, sex cord tumours)
Size
Multiplicity
Rete testis involvement
Pathological stage
Presence of ITGCN
Presence of microvascular invasion
in case of seminoma any non-seminomatour elements.

Prognostic factors for relapse
Seminoma
Size > 4 cm

Rete testis invasion

(If both present relapse rate is 32%, If one present 16% and if none present 12%)

NSGCT
Presence of vascular and lymphatic invasion
Percentage of embryonal carcinoma (>50%)
Proliferation rate (>70%)

If specimen shows seminoma what would you do now?
Complete staging by performing chest abdo/pelvic CT with contrast.
Repeat tumour markers post-op to document kinetics.

Treatment Summary
Seminoma
Stage I
Surveillance or
Chemotherapy

Stage II, III
IIA (Any PT/Tx, N1, Mo, S0-1)
N1 single or multiple lymph node mass <equal 2cm
S1: LDH <1.5XN BhCG<5000 AFP<1000
Either Radiotherapy or
Chemotherapy 3x BEP or 4X EP (If contraindications to Bleomycin)

IIB (Any pT/Tx, N2, Mo, S 0-1)
N2 single or multiple lymph node mass 2-5 cm
S1: LDH <1.5XN BhCG<5000 AFP<1000
Either Chemotherapy
3XBEP or 4XEP (If contraindications to Bleomycin, age>40, smokers)
or Radiotherapy

IIC and higher (Any pT/TX, N3, M0, S0-1)
N3 Lymph node mass > 5 cm in greatest dimension.
Primary chemotherapy according to the same principles used for NSGCT
NSGCT Stage I
(PT1-4/ N0,M0, S0)
Low risk (pT1, No vascular invasion)
Surveillance is standard option
Chemo if conditions against surveillance (not willing)
RPLND if conditions against both surveillance and chemo
High risk (pT2-pT4 vascular invasion present)
Chemo is standard option 1x BEP
NS RPLND if conditions against chemo or
Surveillance also if conditions against chemo
If relapse
3-4 x BEP followed by resection in case of residual tumour
NSGCT Stage II,
Stage IIA (Any PT/Tx, N1, Mo, S0-1) S1
Chemotherapy
PEB X3
If residual tumour
Resection

Stage IIA (Any PT/Tx, N1, Mo, S0-1) S0
Either NS-RPLND
If Pathological stage I
Follow up
If Pathological stage IIA/B
Either follow up or
2 cycles BEP
Or Follow-up after 6 weeks
If Progressive disease
S1
3 X BEP +/- resection of residual tumour
S0
NS-RPLND or
Chemotherapy
If No change
NS-RPLND
If regression
Further follow up

Stage IIC and higher
Good prognosis
Chemotherapy
3X BEP

Intermediate prognosis
4xBEP
Poor prognosis
1x BEP then Tumour markers after 3 weeks
Unfavourable decline
Chemotherapy should be intensified
Favourable decline
BEP x 4
Residual mass after chemo
Surgical resection if visible and markers normal or normalizing.

4.5. Recurrent Urinary Tract Infections

Recurrent urinary tract infections. This could coincide with a stone especially Staghorn calculi so be wary where the station is heading.
Source (Oxford handbook, FRCS viva book)
History taking, examination, clinic based tests, other investigations, management.
Summary:
History:
Find out if it is actual UTI (Positive urine cultures)
Find out if it is recurrent UTIs; twice in six months or three times in 12 months.
Is it persistence? (same organism) or reinfection? (different organisms, 95% of UTIs in females).
Is it complicated UTIs.
Factor that suggest complicated UTI include
Male gender
Elderly
Pregnancy
Indwelling catheter/stent

Recent instrumentation
Immunosuppression
Diabetes
Persistence for more than 7 days
Structurally or functionally abnormal urinary tract.
Ask about sexually transmitted infection (itching, vaginal discharge)
Ask whether the pt is pregnant or takes contraceptive pills if female
Collect all the MSU results, if negative it could be interstitial cystitis (IC), stones, CIS

Ask specifically about risk factors for the development of recurrent UTIs
Reduction of antegrade flow of urine
BOO
Low fluid intake
Neurogenic bladder
Promotion of bacterial colonisation
Sexual intercourse
The use of spermicides
Vaginal oestrogen depletion
Factors facilitating the retrograde ascent of pathogens
Female gender
Indwelling catheter
Urinary/faecal incontinence
Incomplete bladder emptying
Factors that suppress the immunity
Diabetes mellitus
Steroid use
HIV-postivie status
PMH
Diabetes
Stones
Constipation
Neurological illness
Previous UTIs as a child
Family history of UTIs (ABO blood group antigen non-secretors, Lewis non-secretor or P blood group secretors)
Clinical examination
Abdominal examination:
Palpable kidney
Palpable bladder

Loin tenderness
Vaginal examination
Assess tissue oestrogenisation
Genital prolapse
Urethral diverticulum
Focused neurological examination
Investigations:
Urine dipstick
MSU for microscopy, C+S
X-ray KUB
Renal USS + PVR
Management
General advice
High fluid intake
Voiding before and after sexual intercourse
Avoid detergents in the bath
Avoid spermicidal contraceptives (destroys the flora)
Keep urine acidic
Apply topical natural yogurt to vaginal area
Apply topical oestrogen to the vagina
Regular daily intake of cranberry juice
Avoid constipation
Use of antibiotics; three regimes are available
Intermittent self-start therapy as and when needed three days course of quinolone, trimethoprim or nitrofurantoin
Post-intercourse prophylaxis; a single dose of quinolone, trimethoprim, cephalexin or nitrofurantoin immediately after intercourse.
Low dose long-term antibiotic prophylaxis for 6-12 months. Recurrences may be reduced by 95%, however 60% of women develop infections again a few months after stopping the regime.

4.6. Kidney cancer

Scenario
58-year-old man presents with large renal mass on USS. How do you assess?
Full medical history (if symptomatic: 50% haematuria, 40% loin pain, 25% mass, 30% metastatic disease (bone pain, night sweats, fatigue, weight loss, and haemoptysis), less common: pyrexia of unknown origin (9%), acute varicocele due to obstruction of the testicular vein by tumour within the left renal vein (2-5%), lower limb oedema due to venous obstruction. Paraneoplastic syndromes due to ectopic hormone secretion 30%)
Paraneoplastic syndromes: see Figure (2)
Anaemia (30%)
Polycythaemia (5%), due to ectopic erythropoeitin
Hypertension (25%), ectopic renin, renal artery compression
Hypoglycaemia, ectopic insulin
Cushing's syndrome, ectopic ACTH

Hypercalcaemia (10-20%) ectopic PTH-like substance
Gynaecomastia, amenorrhoea, reduced libido, baldness
Stauffer's syndrome: hepatic dysfunction, fever, anorexia

Disease	Renal and other tumours	Gene mutation
Von Hippel–Lindau disease	Clear cell RCC: Clear cell renal cysts	VHL
	Retinal and central nervous system haemangioblastomas, phaeochromocytoma, pancreatic cyst and endocrine tumour, endolymphatic sac tumour, epididymal and broad ligament cystadenomas	
Birt-Hogg-Dubé syndrome	Hybrid oncocytic RCC, chromophobe RCC, oncocytoma, clear cell RCC: multiple and bilateral	Folliculin (FLCN)
	Cutaneous lesions (fibrofolliculoma +++, trichodiscoma, acrochordon), lung cysts, spontaneous pneumothorax, colonic polyps or cancer	
Hereditary papillary RCC	Type 1 papillary RCC: multiple and bilateral	MET
Hereditary leiomyomatosis and RCC	Type 2 papillary RCC: solitary and aggressive	Fumarate hydratase
	Uterine leiomyoma and leiomyosarcoma, cutaneous leiomyoma and leiomyosarcoma	
Tuberous sclerosis complex	Angiomyolipoma, clear cell RCC, cyst, oncocytoma: bilateral and multiple	TSC-1
	Facial angiofibroma, subungual fibroma, hypopigmentation and café au lait spots, cardiac rhabdomyoma, seizure, mental retardation, CNS tubers, lymphangioleiomyomatosis	TSC-2
Familial clear cell RCC	Clear cell RCC	Unknown

Figure (2) Renal cancer syndromes

Risk factors for RCC:
Gender male:female 1.5:1
Age: peak incidence between 60-70
Smoking + tobacco chewing
Renal failure or dialysis
Obesity
Hypertension
Urban dwelling
Low socio-economic status
Occupational asbestos and cadmium
Analgesic phenacetin, thorium dioxide
Sickle cell trait (medullary carcinoma)
Polycystic and horseshoe kidneys.
Genetic:
VHL 50% develop RCC.
Papillary variant of RCC

Birt-Hogg-Dube syndrome (benign tumours of hair follicles, pulmonary cysts, pneumothoraces, renal tumours)

Examination (palpable mass and lymph nodes, a varicocele (for left-sided renal tumours) and lower limb oedema both suggestive of venous involvement.

Investigations: Send blood FBC, ESR, LFTs, Ca, Cr, UEs.

A/P CT scan with IV contrast (>20 Hounsfield units' enhancement is suspicious of malignancy)

Establish morphology of contralateral kidney

Assess extra-renal spread

Assess venous, adrenal, liver and lymph node involvement.

Chest x-ray or a chest CT

MRI scan if there is contrast allergy or renal insufficiency and also useful for assessing IVC involvement.

Doppler ultrasound scan also useful for assessing venous extension.

Bone scan or CT brain for pts with symptoms of metastatic disease.

Prognostic factors for RCC?

TNM Staging system

Fuhrman grade (1-4)

High Fuhrman grade (3,4) is associated with worsening prognosis.

Important: Clear cell tumours have a worse outcome than the chromophobe type, which in turn have a poorer prognosis than the papillary type. The presence of necrosis also confers a poorer prognosis.

Mayo scoring system is widely adopted in the UK and is based on the following criteria: See Table (7)

Feature	Score
Pathologic T stage	
T1a	0
T1b	2
T2	3
T3-4	4
Regional lymph node status	
pNx/Pn0	0
pN1-2	2
Nuclear grading	
G1-2	0
G3	1
G4	3
Tumour size	

<10 cm	0
>10 cm	1
Histologic tumour necrosis	
No	0
Yes	1

Risk group	Score	Estimated metastasis-free survival after 3 years	Estimated metastasis-free survival after 10 years
Low risk	0-2	98%	92.5%
Intermediate risk	3-5	80%	64%
High risk	>6	37%	24%

Table (7): Mayo scoring system
Clinical factors
Cachexia
Poor performance status
Anaemia
Low platelet count

Treatment options:
Indications for adrenalectomy?
Adrenal involvement
Upper pole tumours
T2 cancers greater than 7 cm and multifocal disease.
Indications for nephron sparing surgery?
Absolute indications:
Bilateral synchronous RCC
Anatomical or functional solitary kidney
Relative indications:
Unilateral RCC with a reduced or poorly functioning contralateral kidney
Unilateral RCC in patients with comorbidity associated with potential renal impairment (diabetes, renovascular disease).

Patients with an increased risk of a second renal malignancy (hereditary RCC such as von Hippel-Lindau (VHL) disease).

Elective indications

Localised unilateral RCC with a normal contralateral kidney.

What is the difference in outcome between partial and radical nephrectomy?

Higher risk of local recurrence (5%) and complications (bleeding, urinary leakage) with partial nephrectomy and follow up is more intensive.

Follow up

Low-risk patients will not necessarily require CT follow-up unless they are symptomatic. USS and chest x-ray will suffice.

Intermediate and high risk patients will require an abdominal and pelvic CT and chest imaging for at least 5 years.

Role of nephrectomy in the presence of metastases?

Significantly improve overall survival in patient with metastatic renal cancer treated with interferon immunotherapy. EORTC study showed that median survival with interferon-alpha and nephrectomy (18 months) was significantly better than that with IF-alpha alone (11 months). Similar findings by the SWOG.

What is the role of biopsy in RCC?

Its role will become of increasing importance because

Greater number of small renal masses is being diagnosed

We now have the ability to assess the potential progression of small tumours from novel histological and molecular analyses, which may influence treatment strategies.

Sensitivities and specificities of approximately 90% can be achieved.

Biopsy is not recommended for cystic lesions, or large infiltrative tumours (unless lymphoma is suspected)

Biopsy is not very helpful in the management of oncocytoma due to the difficulty in distinguishing between an oncocytoma and an eosinophilic variant of chromophobe renal-cell cancer and also there is a recognised coexistence of RCC and oncocytoma within the same lesion and at other locations within the kidney.

RCC Scenario

An elderly lady in a haematuria clinic, USS shows possible RCC, the lady was told that she will get a CT scan, however this doesn't happen for three weeks, the patient is concerned and enquires about the delay (communication element).

CT confirms diagnosis and shows possible metastatic disease in the lungs. How to approach? You might get a question about communication in this context (the son is concerned; he phones you and wants to know the results on the phone)

Assess fitness for surgery, offer surgery and repeat chest images in short intervals post-operatively. By adopting this approach, you have offered a possible curative treatment if the lung nodules are not metastatic RCC or in the worst-case scenario cyto-reductive surgery which improves the prognosis of metastatic disease if the lung nodules are indeed metastatic RCC.

Differential diagnosis investigations and management.

Benign: oncocytoma, AML, Cyst. Malignant: RCC or rarely metastatic from another source.

Types of RCC: (FRCS viva book) which ones carry the best or worst prognosis.

Clear cell
Papillary type I, II
Chromophobe

The role of renal biopsy.

See BAUS section below on renal biopsy indications.

Increasingly being used.

Beware of false negative results as biopsy could miss the target tumour area.

BAUS has a nice section on RCC which I include in here (apology for the repetition)

Key questions for the MDT

Tumour/Node/Metastasis (TNM) stage?
Fuhrman grade?
Histological type?
Symptoms?
Risk category (primary or metastatic disease)?
Age?
Co-morbidities?
Life expectancy?
Renal function?
Family history of cancer/renal cancer?

STAGING
OLD AND NEW SYSTEM
See Figure (3)

Tumour stage	TNM 6	TNM 7
T1	≤7 cm; limited to the kidney	≤7 cm; limited to the kidney
T1a	≤4 cm	≤4 cm
T1b	>4 cm	>4 cm
T2	>7 cm; limited to the kidney	>7 cm; limited to the kidney
T2a	NA	>7 cm but <10 cm
T2b	NA	>10 cm
T3	Adrenal or perinephric invasion; involvement of major veins	Perinephric invasion; involvement of major veins
T3a	Perinephric fat or ipsilateral adrenal	Renal vein, perinephric fat
T3b	Renal vein ± vena cava involvement below diaphragm	Vena cava below diaphragm
T3c	Vena cava involvement above diaphragm	Vena cava involvement above diaphragm
T4	Beyond Gerota fascia	Beyond Gerota fascia; ipsilateral adrenal
N1	Single regional lymph node	Single regional lymph node
N2	>1 regional lymph node	>1 regional lymph node

Figure (3): staging of RCC the old and the new system
Assessment and diagnosis
Risk factors for renal cancer

The most well-known risk factors for renal cancer are highlighted below (mentioned earlier)
Age
Peak incidence is at 60-70 years of age
Gender
1.5:1 predominance for men: women
Family history
Having at least 1 first-degree relative with renal cancer increases an individual's relative risk (RR) of renal cancer by 1 to 5 times
The risk is highest if a sibling is affected
The risk of RCC may also be increased in association with a family history of prostate cancer (odds ratio [OR] 1.9), leukaemias (OR 2.2) or any cancer (OR 1.5)
Single gene mutations

Currently there are several renal cancer syndromes, several of which are associated with single gene mutations. Many of these patients will have a family history. These syndromes are outlined in Table 3 below.

Smoking
The RR of RCC for ever-smokers is 1.38 times higher than that for never-smokers
A strong dose-response relationship between number of cigarettes smoked and increased risk of RCC has been established
Smokers with a history of >or equal 20 pack-years have an increased risk of RCC 1.35 times that of never-smokers

Obesity
Increasing body weight and body mass index (BMI) incrementally increases the risk of developing RCC
Being overweight (BMI 25-29.9 kg/m2) increases the risk of RCC by 1.35 times versus BMI <25 kg/m2
Being obese (BMI 30-34.9 kg/m2) increases the risk of RCC by 1.7 times versus BMI <25 kg/m2
Being extremely obese (BMI 35–39.9 kg/m2) increases the risk of RCC by 2.05 times versus BMI <25 kg/m2
Being morbidly obese (BMI > equal 40 kg/m2) increases the risk of RCC by 2.4 times versus BMI <25 kg/m2

Hypertension and anti-hypertensive therapy
The presence of hypertension is estimated to increase the RR of RCC by 1.4--1.9 times compared with normotensive individuals
Systolic blood pressure >160 mmHg increases the RR of RCC by 2.5 times versus <120 mmHg
Diastolic blood pressure >equal100 mmHg increases the RR of RCC by 2.3 times versus <80 mmHg
Treatment with diuretics also increases the risk of RCC (OR 1.43), but this is only significant in women

End-stage renal disease
Patients undergoing dialysis for end-stage renal disease are estimated to have a 3.6 times higher RR of developing renal cancer than healthy individuals

Physical examination
Physical examination has only a limited role in diagnosing RCC, but it may be valuable in cases where any of the following are present:
Palpable abdominal mass
Palpable cervical lymphadenopathy

Non-reducing varicocele
Bilateral lower extremity oedema, suggesting venous involvement
Bony tenderness
Laboratory tests
The most commonly assessed laboratory parameters are:
Serum creatinine concentration
Haemoglobin concentration
Serum alkaline phosphatase concentration
Serum corrected calcium concentration
Plasma C-reactive protein concentration
Serum lactate dehydrogenase concentration

Glomerular filtration rate (GFR) should be measured in patients with:
Compromised renal function
Serum creatinine concentration is elevated
Risk of future renal impairment is increased, e.g. patients with diabetes, chronic pyelonephritis, renovascular, stone or polycystic renal disease
Renal tumour biopsy
Biopsy should be performed in patients with advanced or metastatic disease who are being considered for systemic treatment
Biopsy should be considered in atypical lesions where the diagnosis is not clear and nephrectomy is proposed
Biopsy should be considered in small renal masses where active surveillance or ablative therapy is planned
Ultrasound and computed tomography (CT)
Remember > 20 Hounsfield units' enhancement pre and post contrast is suspicious of cancer.
CT accurately predicts tumour size to within 0.5 cm of the pathological size of the lesion
However, CT also demonstrates a false-positive rate of approximately 10% for the identification of lymph node metastases
In addition, helical CT may identify a requirement for entry into the collecting system for nephron-sparing surgery (NSS)
CT is the most sensitive investigation for the identification of pulmonary metastases
CT helps to establish the morphology of the contralateral kidney, and to assess the primary tumour, extra-renal spread, and venous, adrenal, liver and lymph node involvement.

Evaluation of inferior vena cava tumour thrombus extension can be performed with multi-slice CT, which can produce good coronal reconstructions

Ultrasound is often used for initial screening evaluation when renal disease is suspected. It can be useful to discriminate cystic from solid lesions, to monitor growth of a lesion, and to evaluate lesions found on CT **that are probably hyperdense cysts.**

Detection of small renal lesions with ultrasonography is limited. Lesions <3 cm in diameter are detected only 67% to 79% of the time by conventional ultrasonography.

Bone scans are no longer the standard of care to identify bony metastases – whole body magnetic resonance imaging (MRI) is increasingly used, this is not, however, likely to be routinely available in many centres.

Magnetic resonance imaging

MRI is an option for the evaluation of inferior vena cava tumour thrombus extension and unclassified renal masses (Doppler Ultrasound is also useful in this regard), it can also be indicated if there is contrast allergy or renal insufficiency.

Positron emission tomography (PET)

Currently PET is not a standard investigation in the assessment of renal cancer

it may be useful in detecting distant metastases

Prognostic factors:

Anatomical factors:

TNM Staging.

Histological factors:

As mentioned earlier, High Fuhrman grade is associated with worsening prognosis. Clear cell tumours have a worse outcome than the chromophobe type, which in turn have a poorer prognosis than the papillary type. The presence of necrosis also confers a poorer prognosis.

Clinical factors:

Cachexia, a poor performance status, anaemia and a low platelet count are all associated with higher risk.

Estimated GFR (eGFR) and imaging

Parenteral contrast agents used for CT scanning may cause contrast-induced nephropathy

Those at greatest risk are those with pre-existing renal disease or diabetes

In these patients consider alternative imaging methods

If no alternative, then deploy a reno-protective regimen, including pre-hydration, minimal dose and avoiding repeated doses in a short timeframe

An eGFR of 45 ml/min/1.73m2 is considered to be the threshold at which renoprotective measures should be implemented

Localised disease (T1-T2): Management options: see Figure (4)

Stage T1a
Nephron-sparing surgery if technically possible

Stage T1b
Laparoscopic radical nephrectomy

Consider nephron-sparing surgery if technically feasible or if there is a risk of impaired renal function

Stage T2
Laparoscopic/open radical nephrectomy

Consider nephron-sparing surgery if there is a risk of impaired renal function

Figure (4): management of localised RCC (T1-2)

Management of localised RCC

Surgery

Radical nephrectomy (RN)

There are a number of approaches to performing RN: open and laparoscopic, via either transperitoneal or retroperitoneal access.

Overview

Laparoscopic RN may now be considered a standard of care for patients with T2 and T1b masses not treatable by NSS; but this must ensure:

Early control of the renal blood vessels prior to tumour manipulation

Wide specimen mobilisation external to Gerota's fascia

Avoidance of specimen trauma or rupture

Intact specimen extraction

Routine ipsilateral adrenalectomy is not indicated

Where the adrenal gland appears normal on pre-operative tumour staging (CT, MRI) and intra-operatively where there is no intra-operative suspicion of involvement

Indications for adrenalectomy include an adrenal nodule or an adrenal gland densely adherent to a large upper pole renal tumour. Also indicated for multifocal disease.

Routine extended lymphadenectomy should be restricted to dissection of palpable or enlarged lymph nodes

Patient selection
Stage T1–T2 disease
Normal contralateral kidney
Fitness for surgery/anaesthesia
Baseline GFR >60 ml/min/1.73 m2
In an analysis of data from 1479 patients undergoing RN, those with reduced baseline GFR 45–60 ml/min/1.73 m2 or GFR <45 ml/min/1.73 m2 demonstrated a significant association with lower OS (hazard ratio [HR]: 1.5; p<0.003 and HR: 2.8; p<0.001, respectively)
Absence of co-morbidities
In patients undergoing surgery for RCC, the presence of co-morbidities was associated with worse OS (HR: 1.37; 95% confidence interval [CI]: 1.16–1.63; p=0.0002)

Adverse effects of treatment
Impaired renal function/development of chronic kidney disease and requirement for dialysis
Greater all-cause mortality versus PN

Indications for nephron-sparing surgery:
Absolute:
Bilateral synchronous RCC, and an anatomical or functionally solitary kidney.
Relative:
Unilateral RCC with a reduced or poorly functioning contralateral kidney
Unilateral RCC in patients with comorbidity associated with potential renal impairment (diabetes, renovascular disease(
Patients with an increased risk of a second renal malignancy (hereditary RCC such as von Hippel-Lindau (VHL) disease).
Elective indications
Localised unilateral RCC with a normal contralateral kidney.
RN compared to PN
Worse renal function
Increase all-cause mortality especially in patients < 65

Nephron-sparing surgery/partial nephrectomy
Overview
NSS performed for absolute rather than elective indications has an increased complication rate and higher risk of developing locally recurrent disease, probably due to the larger tumour size

NSS compared with RN is associated with a reduced risk of impaired renal function

Even patients with larger tumours (≤7 cm) who have undergone NSS have achieved outcomes comparable to those following RN

However, for larger tumours follow-up should be intensified due to an increased risk of intrarenal disease recurrence

If the tumour is completely resected, the thickness of the surgical margin does not impact on the likelihood of local recurrence; a minimal tumour-free margin is appropriate to minimise the risk of local recurrence

Laparoscopic PN is an alternative to open NSS for selected patients – the optimal indication is a relatively small and peripheral renal tumour

Potential disadvantages of the laparoscopic approach are the longer warm ischaemia time and increased intraoperative and postoperative complications compared with open surgery

With regard to trans-peritoneal and retro-peritoneal laparoscopic nephrectomy, which is best?

Randomised trials have failed to show a significant advantage for either procedure in terms of blood loss, complication rates and hospital stay.

Retroperitoneal approach might be favoured for

Obese patients

Extensive previous abdominal surgery

Trans-peritoneal route might be favoured for

Anterior or superiorly placed tumour.

Patient selection

Stage T1 disease

Stage T2 disease for absolute indications

Fitness for surgery/anaesthesia

Solitary functional kidney or bilateral disease (absolute indication)

Contralateral kidney with impaired function (relative indication)

Hereditary RCC, with increased risk of future tumours in the contralateral kidney (relative indication)

Normal contralateral kidney (elective indication)

Adverse effects of treatment

Postoperative haemorrhage or urinary leakage

In a randomised trial comparing open PN with open RN for small (≤5 cm), solitary renal tumours, perioperative bleeding ($p<0.001$) and urinary fistulae ($p<0.001$) were significantly more common in the PN group.37 The rate of severe haemorrhage (>1L) was 3.1% after PN and 1.2% after RN. Ten patients (4.4%), all of whom were treated by PN, developed urinary fistulae.

Requirement for repeat intervention

In a randomised trial, the re-operation rate after open PN was 4.4% compared with 2.4% after open RN37

Surveillance following radical nephrectomy

Overview

No RCTs have been published to support specific surveillance measures following RN

There is no consensus regarding the timing of surveillance

Frequency of follow-up is individualised according to the risk of local recurrence or metastasis, assessed using:

Tumour size and extension

Lymph node status

Histological features

Performance status (PS)

Risk scoring systems are recommended for stratifying patients for follow-up, e.g. the Mayo Scoring system. See Figure (5)

In patients considered to be at low risk of relapse (score 0–2), chest X-ray and ultrasound are appropriate assessments

In patients with intermediate (score 3–5) to high risk (score >6) of relapse, CT of the chest and abdomen is recommended as the optimal assessment tool, performed at regular intervals

For patients with intermediate and high risk scores there is no established routine adjuvant therapy

Table 4: Mayo scoring system for prediction of metastases after radical nephrectomy for clear cell carcinoma[57]

Feature	Score
Primary tumour	
pT1a	0
pT1b	2
pT2	3
pT3–pT4	4
Tumour size	
<10 cm	0
≥10 cm	1
Regional lymph node status	
pNx/pN0	0
pN1–pN2	2
Nuclear grade	
1–2	0
3	1
4	3
Tumour necrosis	
Absent	0
Present	1

Figure (5) Mayo scoring for prediction of metastases after radical nephrectomy.
Ablative therapies
Overview
Possible advantages of these techniques include reduced morbidity, outpatient therapy, and the ability to treat patients unsuitable for surgery (open or laparoscopic), including the elderly
Patient selection
Stage T1–T2 disease
Life expectancy >equal 1 year
Small (<5 cm) peripheral (cortical) tumours
Genetic predisposition to multiple tumours
A solitary kidney
Bilateral tumours

Contraindications: irreversible coagulopathies; severe medical instability, e.g. sepsis

Percutaneous radiofrequency ablation (PRFA)
Overview
No RCTs evaluating PFRA in renal cancer have been reported
CT or ultrasound-guided PFRA may be performed under intravenous (IV) sedation and as an outpatient procedure
Assessment of treatment success is performed using CT scanning or MRI

Patient selection
Tumours <5.5 cm, in situations where surgery is not feasible
Single functioning kidney
Normal contralateral kidney
Multifocal RCC

Adverse effects of treatment
The most commonly reported complication associated with PRFA is haematoma development
The frequency of this has been reported as ranging from 4% to 8% of patients
Haemorrhage has been reported in 6% of patients60
Urinary obstruction has been reported in 4–10% of patients
In a series of 24 patients, 2 experienced colonic injuries following PFRA
A meta-analysis of data from 99 studies and including 6471 tumours has recently been published
When compared with NSS, PFRA was associated with an RR of 18.23 and cryoablation an RR of 7.45 for local disease progression

Cryoablation
Overview
No RCTs evaluating cryoablation in renal cancer have been reported
Defining RFS is variable because post-ablation biopsies are not commonly performed and interpretation of post-ablation cross-sectional imaging can be difficult
Recent changes and advancements in probe technology make percutaneous treatment easier than open or laparoscopic techniques

Adverse effects of treatment
In a study involving 27 cryoablation treatments, 1 episode of haemorrhage occurred, which required a blood transfusion and 1 patient experienced an abscess

in an analysis of 48 cases (49 tumours), percutaneous cryoablation was performed under sedation and as an outpatient procedure

At a mean follow-up of 1.6 years, for patients with RCC, 11% were considered to be treatment failures

Surveillance

A meta-analysis of 880 patients with 936 renal masses demonstrated that only 18 progressed to metastasis at a mean of 40 months

A subset of these patients with individual data shows that the mean diameter was small at 2.3 ± 1.3 cm, mean linear growth rate was 0.31 ± 0.38 cm per year at a mean follow-up of 33.5 ± 22.6 months

Sixty-five masses (23%) exhibited zero net growth under surveillance, and none of those masses progressed to metastasis

A pooled analysis revealed that older age, larger tumour volume and a more rapid growth rate were associated with progression

Surgery
Surgical management of T3–T4 disease. See Figure (6)

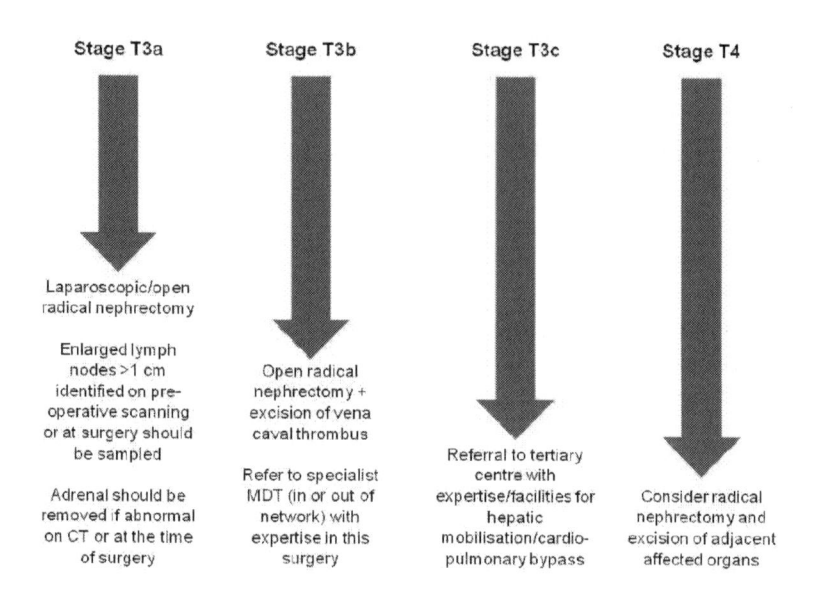

Stage T3a	Stage T3b	Stage T3c	Stage T4
Laparoscopic/open radical nephrectomy	Open radical nephrectomy + excision of vena caval thrombus	Referral to tertiary centre with expertise/facilities for hepatic mobilisation/cardio-pulmonary bypass	Consider radical nephrectomy and excision of adjacent affected organs
Enlarged lymph nodes >1 cm identified on pre-operative scanning or at surgery should be sampled	Refer to specialist MDT (in or out of network) with expertise in this surgery		
Adrenal should be removed if abnormal on CT or at the time of surgery			

Figure (6) Surgical management of T3-4 disease

Surgical management of T3-T4 disease
Radical nephrectomy
Overview
About 5–10% of RCCs extend into the venous system as tumour thrombi, often ascending the inferior vena cava as high as the right atrium
RN is strongly indicated for locally advanced RCC
Total surgical excision should be the objective of surgery, presuming the patient is an appropriate candidate and vital structures are not compromised
RN will occasionally require en bloc resection of adjacent organs, isolation and temporary occlusion of the regional vasculature, and venous thrombectomy
Patient selection
Stage T3–T4 disease (involvement of adrenal gland and/or renal vasculature) or metastatic disease
PS 0–1

In 601 patients with T2–T3b RCC, 567 underwent RN and 34 underwent NSS81
After a mean follow-up of 43.4 months, disease recurred in 28.9% receiving RN and 12.0% of patients receiving NSS
A retrospective analysis of 38 patients with T3–T4 disease evaluated RN and resection of adjacent organ or structure resection82
34 patients (90%) had died from their disease after a median of 11.7 months after surgery
In an analysis of data from 11,182 patients with metastatic RCC, those who underwent RN experienced a significantly longer median OS than those who did not undergo surgery (11 versus 4 months; p<0.001)83
The survival benefit was similar regardless of age, race and gender

Cytoreductive nephrectomy
CN has been suggested to reduce the total burden of disease in patients with metastatic RCC, increasing the time before tumour burden becomes lethal
However, the benefit of CN is supported by evidence from the era of IFN-α and cannot automatically be extrapolated into the modern era in combination with targeted molecules

Patient selection
Good PS with adequate cardiac and pulmonary function
WHO PS 0 or 1
In a retrospective analysis of data from 418 patients undergoing CN, those with an Eastern Co-operative Oncology Group (ECOG) PS 2 or 3 experienced a median DSS of 6.6 months compared with 27 months and 13.8 months in patients with ECOG PS 0 and 1, respectively

Fit for surgery
>75% of tumour burden in the involved kidney
Solitary brain or liver metastases
Patient acceptance of the procedure after full discussion of risks and benefits
Adjuvant tumour cell-derived vaccines

Clinical evidence
In 89 patients with T3/N0/M0 disease, administration of an autologous tumour cell lysate

vaccine following RN was associated with a greater PFS rate than no adjuvant therapy (74.4% versus 65.9%)

Adjuvant immunotherapy

309 patients were randomised to adjuvant IL-2, interferon-alpha (IFN-α) and 5-fluorouracil (5-FU) in patients with a high risk of relapse after nephrectomy for RCC

There were no statistically significant differences between the two arms in terms of DFS or OS

Interferon alpha doesn't significantly improve overall response, time to progression, OS, DFS.

Resection of metastases

Patients with limited metastatic disease can be considered for metastasectomy

Patient selection

Good PS

Resectable, residual metastases following previous response to immunotherapy

Patients who relapse with oligometastatic disease >1 year are more likely to benefit from metastatectomy than those who relapse <1 year post-nephrectomy

The decision to proceed with metastatectomy should be taken after a test of time to exclude as far as possible those patients who are rapidly relapsing with metastatic disease appearing at other sites

A minimum 3-month period is recommended

Systemic therapy

In patients with metastatic RCC for whom no surgical options are advisable, systemic therapy should be considered

Although several active agents are now available for the treatment of metastatic disease, their general inability to produce durable CRs necessitates chronic treatment in most patients

The benefits must therefore be weighed against the overall burden of treatment, including acute and chronic toxicity, time and cost58

Immunotherapy (interferon-alpha and interleukin-2)

Overview

IFN-α is a treatment option for selected patients with a good prognosis

IL-2 is not recommended as a routine treatment as there is a lack of Level 1 evidence proving a survival advantage

High-dose IL-2 may be an option for carefully selected patients referred to experienced centres

Adverse effects of treatment
The most common AEs associated with IFN-α and IL-2 therapy are hypotension, nausea, vomiting, diarrhoea and anaemia

Patient selection
Good PS (ECOG 0 or 1)
Good renal, hepatic and haematological function
No cardiac or central nervous system disorders
No active infections

Angiogenesis inhibitors
Overview
Patients should preferably undergo biopsy prior to the initiation of treatment with these agents

Sunitinib (TKI inhibitor)
Patient selection
Good and intermediate prognostic groups according to MSKCC criteria125
Clear cell histology
Adequate cardiac and renal function
No recent or planned surgery
In the Phase III study, **the most common AEs** reported in the sunitinib group included leukopenia (78% of patients), neutropenia (72%), anaemia (71%), increased serum creatinine concentration (66%), thrombocytopenia (65%), diarrhoea (53%) and fatigue (51%)
In the subsequent Phase III trial, 750 patients with previously untreated metastatic RCC were randomised to 6-week cycles of oral sunitinib (50 mg once-daily for 4 weeks, followed by 2 weeks off) or SC IFN-α (9 million units 3 times per week)
Median PFS was 11 months in patients receiving sunitinib and 5 months in patients receiving IFN-α (HR: 0.42; 95%CI: 0.32–0.54; $p<0.001$)

Pazopanib (TKI inhibitor)
Patient selection
Good and intermediate prognostic groups according to MSKCC criteria125
Clear cell histology
Adequate cardiac and renal function
No recent or planned surgery

Adverse effects of treatment
mucositis/stomatitis, hypothyroidism and hand-foot syndrome

arterial thromboembolic events
elevation of alanine aminotransferase
elevation of aspartate aminotransferase.
Temsirolimus (m-TOR inhibitor)
Patient selection
Good PS (Karnofsky score ≥60)
Good renal, hepatic and haematological function
At least 3 of 6 predictors of short survival
Adverse effects of treatment
rash (47% of patients), anaemia (45%), nausea (37%), anorexia (32%), pain (28%) and dyspnoea (28%)
National Institute for Health and Clinical Excellence (NICE) Technology Appraisal Guidance
NICE has reviewed a number of systemic therapies for the treatment of advanced/metastatic RCC
First-line therapy
Sunitinib is recommended as first-line therapy in patients with metastatic RCC who are suitable for immunotherapy and have an ECOG PS of 0 or 1
Pazopanib is recommended as a first-line treatment option for people with advanced renal cell carcinoma:
Who have not received prior cytokine therapy and have an ECOG PS of 0 or 1 and
If the manufacturer provides pazopanib with a 12.5% discount on the list price, and provides a possible future rebate linked to the outcome of the head-to-head COMPARZ trial, as agreed under the terms of the patient access scheme and to be confirmed when the COMPARZ trial data are made available
Bevacuzimab, sorafenib and temsirolimus are not recommended as first-line treatment options for patients with metastatic RCC

Second-line therapy
Sorafenib and sunitinib are not recommended as second-line treatment options for patients with metastatic RCC129
Palliative care
Surgery
Overview
Nephrectomy may be used to resolve symptoms such as pain and bleeding arising from the primary tumour
Tumour embolisation
Overview

This approach may be considered in patients with large tumours that cannot be resected and that are causing overt symptoms

Common side effects include fever and transient pain, but these can usually be managed with non-steroidal anti inflammatory drugs

Palliative radiotherapy

Overview

This is an option for patients with large tumours with bleeding where no other options are feasible or available

In addition, radiotherapy of bone metastases from RCC can provide short-term pain relief

4.7. Kidney Stones

Non-infection stones
• Calcium oxalate
• Calcium phosphate
• Uric acid
Infection stones
• Magnesium ammonium phosphate
• Carbonate apatite
• Ammonium urate
Genetic causes
• Cystine
• Xanthine
• 2,8-dihydroxyadenine
Drug stones

Figure (7) Different types of stones

I include here also the EAU guidelines which are also useful in this regard.

Aetiology and classification:

Stone incidence depends on geographical, climatic, ethnic, dietary and genetic factors.

In countries with a high standard of life such as Sweden, Canada or the US, renal stone prevalence is notably high (> 10%).

Stones can be classified into

Infection and non-infection stones

Genetic stones

Drug stones. See Figure (7)

Risk groups for stone formation

50% of recurrent stone formers have just one lifetime recurrence

Highly recurrent disease is observed in slightly more than 10% of patients

High risk stone formers

General factors

Early onset (Children and teenagers)

Familial Hx

Brushite-containing stones (CaHPO4.2H2O)

Uric acid stones

Infection stones

Solitary kidney (Prevention here is more important)

Diseases associated with stone formation
Hyperparathyroidism
Metabolic syndrome
Nephrocalcinosis
Polycystic kidney disease (PKD)
Gastrointestinal diseases (i.r. Jejuno-ileal bypass, intestinal resection, Crohn's disease,
malabsorptive conditions, enteric hyperoxaluria after urinary diversion) and bariatric surgery
Sarcoidosis
Spinal cord injury, neurogenic bladder
Genetically determined stone formation
Cystinuria (Type A, B and AB)
Primary hyperoxaluria (PH)
Renal tubular acidosis (RTA) type I
2,8 - Dihydroxyadeninuria
Xanthinuria
Lesch-Nyhan syndrome
Cystic fibrosis
Drugs associated with stone formation
Anatomical abnormalities associated with stone formation
Medually sponge kidney (tubular ectasia)
Ureteropelvic junction (UPJ) obstruction
Calyceal diverticulum, calyceal cyst
Ureteral stricture
Vesico-uretero-renal reflux
Horseshoe kidney
Ureterocele
Classification of stones
Stone size
up to 5 mm
5-10 mm
10-20 mm
>20 mm
Stone location
Upper, middle or lower calyx
Renal pelvis
Upper, middle or distal ureter
Urinary bladder

X-ray characteristics

Radiopaque
Calcium oxalate dihydrate
Calcium oxalate monohydrate
calcium phosphates

Poor radiopacity
Magnesium ammonium phosphate
Apatite
Cystine

Radiolucent
Uric acid
Ammonium urate
Xanthine
2,8 - Dihydroxyadenine
Drug-stones

Diagnostic evaluation
Hx and examination

Presentation

Ureteric stones
Loin pain, vomiting and sometimes fever. Or asymptomatic

Diagnostic imaging

Uss
Primary diagnostic imaging tool
Safe, reproducible and inexpensive
Sensitivity of 45% and specificity of 94% for ureteric stones
Sensitivity of 45% and specificity of 88% for renal stones

KUB
Sensitivity of 44-77% and specificity of 80-87%

Recommendation
With fever or solitary kidney, and when diagnosis is doubtful, immediate imaging is indicated

Evaluation of patients with acute flank pain/suspected ureteral stones
NCCT (Non contrast CT) is standard and replaced IVU. (more accurate)
Following initial US assessment, use NCCT to confirm stone diagnosis in patients with acute flank pain, because it is superior to IVU.
NCCT detects uric acid and xanthine stones (radiolucent) but not indinavir stones

Info obtained from NCCT
Stone density

Stone Inner structure
Skin to stone distance
Surrounding anatomy

Disadvantages of CT
No info on renal function and urinary collecting system anatomy
Higher radiation dose
This can be reduced by Low dose CT
Sensitivity of 86% for ureteric stones < 3mm
Sensitivity of 100% for > 3mm
Meta-analysis showed that LDCT has Pooled sensitivity 96.6% and specificity of 94.9%

Recommendation for radiologic examinations of patients with acute flank pain/suspected ureteric stones.
Following initial USS assessment, use NCCT to confirm stone diagnosis in patients with acute flank pain, as it is superior to IVU.

Radiation exposure of imaging modalities

X-ray KUB	0.5-1	mSv
X-ray chest	0.05- 0.1	mSv
IVU	1.3-3.5	mSv
Regular dose NCCT	4.5-5	mSv (100 chest x-ray)
Low-dose NCCT	0.97-1.9	mSv
Enhanced CT	25-35	mSv (500 chest x-ray)

Recommendations for radiologic examination of patients with renal stones
Perform a contrast study if stone removal is planned and the anatomy of the renal collecting system needs to be assessed.
Use enhanced CT in complex cases because it enables 3D reconstruction of the collecting system, as well as measurement of stone density and skin-to-stone distance. IVU may also be used.

Diagnostics - metabolism – related
Recommendations
Urine
Dipstick test of spot urine sample (RCC, WCC, nitrite, pH)
Microscopy
Blood
Creatinine

Uric acid
(Ionised) calcium
Sodium
Potassium
Blood cell count
CRP
Perform a coagulation test (PTT and INR) if intervention is likely or planned.
If no intervention is planned Na, K, CRP, Coag are not needed.
Easiest means of diagnosis is analysing a passed stone

Recommendations
Perform stone analysis in first-time formers using a valid procedure (XRD or IRS)
Repeat stone analysis in patients
Presenting with recurrent stones despite drug therapy
With early recurrence after complete stone clearance
With late recurrence after a long stone-free period because stone composition may change

Diagnosis for Special groups/conditions:
Pregnancy
X-ray in the first trimester should be reserved for patients in which alternative imaging methods have failed
USS Primary diagnostic tool for pregnant patients with suspected renal colic.
MRI can be used as a second-line procedure (level of obstruction, visualise stone)
Low dose CT last-line option

Recommendations
Use ultrasound as the preferred method of imaging in pregnant women
In pregnant women, use MRI as a second-line imaging modality
In pregnant women, use low-dose CT as a last-line option
Treat all non-complicated cases of urolithiasis in pregnancy conservatively (except those that have clinical indications for intervention)
If intervention becomes necessary, place a ureteral stent or a percutaneous nephrostomy tube as readily available primary options
Use ureteroscopy as a reasonable alternative to avoid long-term stenting/drainage.

In case of stent insertion ensure regular follow-up until final stone removal because of the higher encrustation tendency of stents during pregnancy.

Management of stones in patients with urinary diversion:
Perform PCNL to remove large renal stones in patients with urinary diversion, as well as for ureteral stones that cannot be accessed via a retrograde approach or that are not amenable to ESWL.

Management of stones in transplanted kidneys
Perform US or NCCT to rule out calculi in patients with transplanted kidneys, unexplained fever, or unexplained failure to thrive (particularly in children)

Offer patients with transplanted kidneys, any of the contemporary treatment modalities, including shockwave therapy, (flexible) ureteroscopy, and percutaneous nephrolithotomy as management options.

Complete metabolic evaluation after stone removal.

Children
Considered high risk
In paediatric patients, the most common non-metabolic disorders facilitating stone formation are VUR, PUJ Obstruction, neurogenic bladder and other voiding difficulties.

Recommendations
In all paediatric patients, complete a metabolic evaluation based on stone analysis
Collect stone material for analysis to classify the stone type

Diagnostic imaging in children
The principle of ALARA (As Low as Reasonably Achievable) should be observed.

Ultrasound
Primary technique

Advantages
no radiation
no need for anaesthesia
Colour Doppler US shows differences in the ureteric jet and resistive index of the arciform arteries of both kidneys, which are indicative of the grade of obstruction

Disadvantages
Fails to identify stones in >40% of paediatric patients
Provides limited info on renal function

X-ray KUB
IVU
Same radiation dose as voiding cystourethrography (0.33mSV)
Helical CT
NCCT detects 95% of stones in children
MRU
No good for stones, but it provides
Detailed anatomical information of the collecting system,
The location of an obstruction or stenosis in the ureter and
Renal parenchymal morphology
Recommendations
In children, use ultrasound as first-line imaging modality when a stone is suspected; it should include the kidney, fluid-filled bladder and the ureter next to the kidney and the (filled bladder)
If US does not provide the required information, perform a KUB radiography (or low-dose NCCT)
Collect stone material for analysis to classify the stone type.
In all paediatric patients, complete a metabolic evaluation based on stone analysis as they have a high risk of recurrence.
In children, perform PCNL for the treatment of renal pelvic or caliceal stones with a diameter > 20mm
For intracorporeal lithotripsy, use the same devices as in adults (Ho:YAG laser, pneumatic- and US lithotripters)
Disease management
Acute treatment of a patient with renal colic
Pain relief
NSAIDs including metamizole (dipyrone) a pyrazolone NSAID are effective and better than opioids.
Diclofenac and ibuprofen increase major coronary events
Diclofenac is contraindicated in pts with CHF, IHD, PVD, CVD.
Pethidine is associated with high rate of vomiting
Prevention of recurrent renal colic
If stone is expected to pass spontaneously NSAID or suppositories help.
Diclofenac can affect renal function if there is an impairment already.
Daily alpha-blockers might reduce recurrent colic
If analgesia fails medically, stent, nephrostomy or stone removal should be performed.
Recommendations
Provide immediate pain relief in acute stone episodes.

Whenever possible, offer an NSAID as the first drug of choice. e.g. metamizol (dipyrone); alternatively, depending on cardio-vascular risk factors diclofenac, indomethacin or ibuprofen

Offer hydromorphine, pentazocine or tramadol as a second choice

Use alpha-blockers to reduce recurrent colic in informed pts

for symptomatic ureteral stones, urgent stone removal as first-line treatment is a feasible option in selected cases

Management of sepsis and/or anuria in obstructed kidney
Urological emergency
Urgent decompression is often necessary

Two options

Stent

Nephrostomy

No good-quality evidence to suggest that ureteric stenting has more complications than nephrostomy

Definitive stone removal should be delayed until the infection is cleared following a course of abx.

In children stents have some advantages compared to PCN in case of acute anuria.

For decompression of the renal collecting system, ureteral stents and percutaneous nephrostomy catheters are equally effective.

Be aware, these are EAU guidelines, however in the UK and generally speaking nephrostomies are the preferred choice in septic patients. And in the interview examiners will expect you to justify that and tell the difference between the two.

Briefly, the advantages of nephrostomy are:

Reduces the pressure in the kidney,

Drains the pus,

Avoids ureteric injury/manipulation,

Avoids general anaesthetic,

Allows monitoring of urine output straight from kidney, allows access for subsequent intervention if required.

The advantages of stent are:

No need for radiologist,

Less risk of injury to adjacent organs,

No need for an outer bag.

Recommendations

Urgently decompress the collecting system in case of sepsis with obstructing stones, using percutaneous drainage or ureteral stenting

Delay definitive treatment of the stone until sepsis is resolved.

Further measures
Urine and blood cultures
Start Abx immediately (regimen re-evaluated in light of the culture test)
ITU might become necessary

Recommendations
Collect (again) urine for antibiogram test following decompression
Start antibiotics immediately (+ ITU if necessary)
Re-evaluate antibiotic regimen following antibiogram findings.

Observation of ureteral stones
In patients with newly diagnosed small ureteral stones, if active stone removal is not indicated, observe patient initially along with periodic evaluation
Offer patients appropriate medication to facilitate stone passage during observation.

Observation of kidney stones:
It is still debatable whether kidney stones should be treated, or whether annual follow-up is sufficient for asymptomatic caliceal stones that have remained stable for 6 months.
Follow-up periodically in cases where renal stones are not treated (initially after 6 months and yearly follow-up of symptoms and stone status (US, KUB or CT))
Assess comorbidity, stone composition if possible and patient preference when making treatment decisions

Medical expulsive therapy (MET)
Patients who elect for an attempt at spontaneous passage or MET should have well-controlled pain, no clinical evidence of sepsis, and adequate renal functional reserve.
Offer alpha-blockers as MET as one of the options
Counsel patients regarding the lack of efficacy in a recent large multicentre trial, attendant risks of MET, including associated drug side effects as well as inform the patients that alpha-blockers are administered off-label
Follow up patients in short intervals to monitor stone position and assess for hydronephrosis.

Pharmacological treatment
Percutaneous irrigation chemolysis
an option for infection and uric acid stones (rarely used). for dissolution of struvite stones, Suby's G solution (10% hemiacidrin; pH 3.5-4) can be used
Oral chemolysis

Uric acid stones can be dissolved by oral chemolysis.
Oral chemolitholysis is based on alkalinisation of urine (alkaline citrate or sodium bicarbonate)
The pH should be 7.0 - 7.2
Higher pH risk calcium phosphate stone formation
US could be used to monitor radiolucent stones during therapy (NCCT might be necessary)
Tamsulosin + alkalinisation achieves the highest stone free rates for distal uric acid ureteral stones

Recommendations
Inform the patient how to modify the dosage of alkalising medication according to urine pH, which has a direct consequence of such medication
Inform the patient how to monitor urine pH by dipstick three times a day (at regular intervals). Morning urine must be included
Carefully monitor radiolucent stones during/after therapy
Inform the patient of the significance of compliance

SWL
Success depends on
Efficacy of lithotripter and size/location and composition of stone
Patient's habitus
Performance of SWL

Contraindications of SWL
Pregnancy
Bleeding diatheses
Uncontrolled UTIs
Severe skeletal malformations and severe obesity
Arterial aneurysm in the vicinity
Anatomical obstruction distal to the stone

Stenting in ESWL
Stent doesn't improve SFR
Reduces risk of renal colic and obstruction but not steinstrasse or infection
Do not routinely use a stent as part of SWL treatment of ureteral stones

Pacemaker in SWL
SWL is ok.

Defibrillators in ESWL
Firing mode temporarily reprogrammed during SWL (this might not be necessary with new-generation lithotripters)

SW rate

Lowering from 120 to 60-90 shock waves/min improves SFR
Tissue damage increases with frequency
Use a shock wave frequency of 1.0-1.5 Hz.
Number of shock waves, energy setting and repeat treatment sessions
No consensus on the maximum number of shock waves
Animal studies showed better SFRs using stepwise power ramping.
No conclusive data on intervals between sessions. Sessions are feasible within 1 day for ureteral stones
Clinical experience has shown that repeat sessions are feasible (within 1 day for ureteral stones)
Improvement of acoustic coupling
Proper acoustic coupling between the cushion of the treatment head and the patients' skin is important. USS gel is the most widely used lithotripsy coupling agent
Ensure correct use of the coupling agent because this is crucial for effecive shock wave transportation

Procedural control
Better results by experienced clinicians. Careful imaging control of localisation leads to better outcomes
Maintain careful fluoroscopic and/or ultrasonographic monitoring during the procedure
Pain control
Use proper analgesia because it improves treatment results by limiting induced movements and excessive respiratory excursions.
Prescribe antibiotics prior to ESWL in the case of infected stones or bacteriuria.

Steinstrasse
Steinstrasse accumulation of stone fragments in ureter. 4-7% of cases of SWL (Stone size is major factor)
Can cause silent ureteric obstruction in 23% of cases
insertion of stent before SWL in stones > 15 mm can be preventative
Conservative treatment is an initial option if asymptomatic
MET reduces the need for intervention
MET increases the stone expulsion rate of steinstrasse
When spontaneous passage is unlikely, further treatment of steinstrasse is indicated
SWL is indicated in asymptomatic and symptomatic cases, with no evidence of UTI, when large stone fragments are present

Ureteroscopy is effective for the treatment of steinstrasse
placement of PCN tube or ureteral stent is indicated for symptomatic ureteric obstruction with/wihout UTI.

Recommendations
Treat steinstrasse associated with urinary tract infection/fever preferably with percutaneous nephrostomy
Treat steinstrasse when large stone fragments are present with SWL or ureterorenoscopy

PCNL:
Preoperative imaging:
Perform preprocedural imaging, including contrast medium where possible or retrograde study when starting the procedure, to assess stone comprehensiveness and anatomy of the collecting system to ensure safe access to the renal stone.

Intracorporeal lithotripsy:
Use ultrasonic, ballistic and Ho:YAG devices for intracorporeal lithotripsy during PCNL.
When using flexible instruments, use the Ho;YAG laser since it is currently the most effective device.

Nephrostomy and stents after PCNL:
In uncomplicated cases, perform a tubeless (no nephrostomy tube) or totally tubeless (no nephrostomy tube and no ureteral stent) PCNL procedure as it is a safe alternative.

Uretero-renoscopy (URS)
Place a safety wire
Do not perform stone extraction using a basket without endoscopic visualisaiton of the stone (blind basketing)
Use Ho:YAG laser lithotripsy for (flexible) URS.
In uncomplicated cases there is no need to insert a stent

Open and laparoscopic surgery:
Offer laparoscopic or open surgical stone removal in rare cases in which SWL, (flexible) URS and PCNL fail, or are unlikely to be successful.
When expertise is available, perform surgery laparoscopically before proceeding to open surgery, especially when the stone mass is centrally located.
For ureterolithotomy, perform laparoscopy for large impacted stones when endoscopic lithotripsy or ESWL has failed.

Indication for active stone removal and selection of procedure:
Ureter:

Stones with a low likelihood of spontaneous passage
Persistent pain despite adequate pain medication
Persistent obstruction
Renal insufficiency (renal failure, bilateral obstruction, single kidney)
Kidney:
Stone growth
Stones in high-risk patients for stone formation
Obstruction caused by stones
Infection
Symptomatic stones (e.g. pain, haematuria)
Stones >15 mm
Stones <15 mm if observation is not the option of choice
Patient preference
Comorbidity
Social situation of the patient (e.g. profession or travelling)
Choice of treatment
Stone removal:
General recommendations:
Obtain a urine culture or perform urinary microscopy before any treatment is planned. Exclude or treat UTIs prior to endourologic stone removal.
Offer peri-operative antibiotic prophylaxis to all patients undergoing endourological treatment.
Offer active surveillance to patients at high-risk for thrombotic complications in the presence of an asymptomatic caliceal stone
Decide on temporary discontinuation, or bridging of antithrombotic therapy in high-risk patients, in consultation with the internist.
Perform retrograde (flexible) ureterorenoscopy if stone removal is essential and antithrombotic therapy cannot be discontinued, since it is associated with less morbidity.
The following are at elevated risk of haemorrhage
ESWL
PCNL
PCN
Laparoscopic surgery
Open surgery
If uncorrected bleeding disorder or continued antithrombotic therapy, URS is better than SWL/PNL
Risk stratification for bleeding
Low-risk bleeding procedures

Cystoscopy (Flexi)
Ureteral catheterization
Extraction of ureteric stent
Ureteroscopy

Management of patients with residual fragments

Identify biochemical risk factors and appropriate stone prevention in patients with residual fragments or stones.

Follow-up patients with residual fragments or stones regularly to monitor disease course

After ESWL and URS, and in the presence of residual fragments, offer MET using an alpha-blocker to improve fragment clearance.

Metabolic evaluation and recurrence prevention
General advice

Fluid intake: fluid amount: 2.5 – 3.0 L/day

Circadian drinking, Neutral ph beverages, Diuresis > 2.5L/day, specific weight of urine: <1010

Nutritional advice for a balanced diet: balanced diet, rich in vegetables and fibre, normal calcium content: 1-1.2g/day, limited NaCl content 4-5g/day, limited animal protein content: 0.8-1.0 g/kg/day

Lifestyle advice to normalize general risk factors: BMI retain a normal BMI level, Adequate physical activity, Balancing of excessive fluid loss.

Metabolic intervention according to abnormality

Urinary risk factor	Suggest treatment
Hypercalciuria	Thiazide + potassium citrate
Hyperoxaluria	Oxalate restriction
Enteric hyperoxaluria	Potassium citrate Calcium supplement Diet reduced in fat and oxalate
Hypocitraturia	Potassium citrate
Hypocitraturia	Sodium bicarobonate if intolerant to potassium citrate
Hyperuricosuria	Allopurinol Febuxostat
High sodium excretion	Restricted intake of salt
Small urine volume	Increased fluid intake
Urea level indicating a high	Avoid excessive intake of

| intake of animal protein | animal protein |
| No abnormality identified | High fluid intake |

Important topics in stone disease:
Staghorn calculi:
Investigations:
Urine (C+S)
Blood (FBC, UEs, Ca, urate)
Urine spot test for cystine.
CT or IVU (Define stone burden and calyceal anatomy)
99mTc DMSA Renogram (to assess split renal function prior to planning definitive treatment)

What is DMSA (Dimercaptosuccinic acid) (Important)?
DMSA is a protein that is actively extracted and bound by functioning renal tubules, with very little filtered. Images are taken 2-3 hours later with a gamma camera.

Kidney Stones:
Treatment options for staghorn calculi in an elderly unfit patient or in an otherwise fit patient. (FRCS viva book is very good in this regard) (Important)

Should we treat staghorn calculi?
Blandy and Singh paper is most frequently quoted. They concluded that there is no such clinical entity as a "silent staghorn", based on the post-mortem study. Long term survival is better in those treated surgically (mortality rate of 7%) than in those managed conservatively (mortality rate of 28%).

Teichman paper further supported Blandy and Singh paper. It demonstrated that no patient with complete clearance of fragments died of renal related causes, compared with 3% of those without clearance of fragments and **67%** of those who refused treatment. Overall rate of renal deterioration was 100% in those who refused treatment compared to 28% in those who accepted treatment.

What are the indications and contraindications for PCNL?
Indications:
Stone size:
Stones > 3 cm in diameter
Renal pelvis stones > 2 cm in diameter

Lower pole stones > 1 cm in diameter
Staghorn stones
Presence of Obstruction (ESWL is contraindicated)
Anatomical considerations:
Horseshoe kidney, calyceal diverticular stones, kyphoscoliosis or obesity
Failed ESWL/URS
Stones associated with a foreign body
Patient choice

Contraindications for PCNL:
Absolute
Uncorrected bleeding disorder
Pregnancy
Sepsis
Poor kidney function (< 15%) where nephrectomy would be indicated
Need for coincidental open procedure

Relative:
Horseshoe or ectopic kidney (high risk of bowel injury)
Medical problems (high anaesthetic risk)
Anterior calyceal diverticulum.

Consenting for the procedure:
Complications:

Complications related to access:
Bleeding
Blood transfusion (11%)
Embolization (1%)
Nephrectomy (rare)
Perforation of adjacent organs (bowel < 1%, pneumothorax 0-5%)
Access failure (5%)

What are the treatment options for staghorn calculi? (Important)

PCNL (if infundibula is narrow) (highest success rate)
ESWL (if infundibula is large) +- Stent or nephrostomy to achieve renal drainage
PCNL + ESWL
Open surgery (nephrolithotomy, pyelolithotomy) (significant co-morbidity)
Ureteroscopy (limited use)
Conservative in unfit patients

Don't forget medical therapy (urease inhibitors) AHA (Acetohydroxamic acid) + antibiotics.

Lower pole renal calculus:
1.4 cm stone in right lower pole what are the treatment options?
Treatment options:
ESWL
PCNL
Flexible URS
Two famous studies lower pole study I, and lower pole study II compared ESWL and PCNL as well as ESWL and URS respectively.

Lower pole study I:
For stone size between < 10mm – 21-30mm: Overall 3-month stone-free rates were 95% for PCNL and 37% for ESWL. PCNL has higher complication rates(23% versus 12%), Both are equally effective for stones less than 10 mm in diameter (63% PCNL versus 63% ESWL), and PCNL was more cost-effective for larger stones. **The conclusions of this study is** PCNL should be regarded as the primary approach for LPS larger than 10 mm.

Lower pole study II:
For stone size <10mm no statistically significant difference in stone-free rates were found between ESWL and URS for LPS even though URS was 15% better. A different outcome might be achieved if such a study were to be repeated. (More advanced technology and larger number of patients)
URS should be primary approach for patients with LPS who failed ESWL as the success rate is 86% for LPS larger than 20mm in diameter.
Therefore ESWL is the preferred initial approach for most patients with LPS smaller than 1 cm, as it is a less invasive approach, and does not require GA. If ESWL fails then either URS or PCNL could be considered as alternatives.

Ureteric Stones:
For proximal ureteric stones, it appears that ESWL may be superior for stones <10mm in diameter, but URS is better for stones > 10 mm.
For distal ureteric stones, URS is considered to be superior irrespective of size.
For mid-ureteric stones, the treatments are generally considered to be equivalent.
EAU Guidelines:

EAU have slightly different recommendations when it comes to kidney and ureteric stones. Figure (8,9). ESWL is equal to URS for proximal ureteric stones <10mm and also equal to URS for distal ureteric stones <10mm

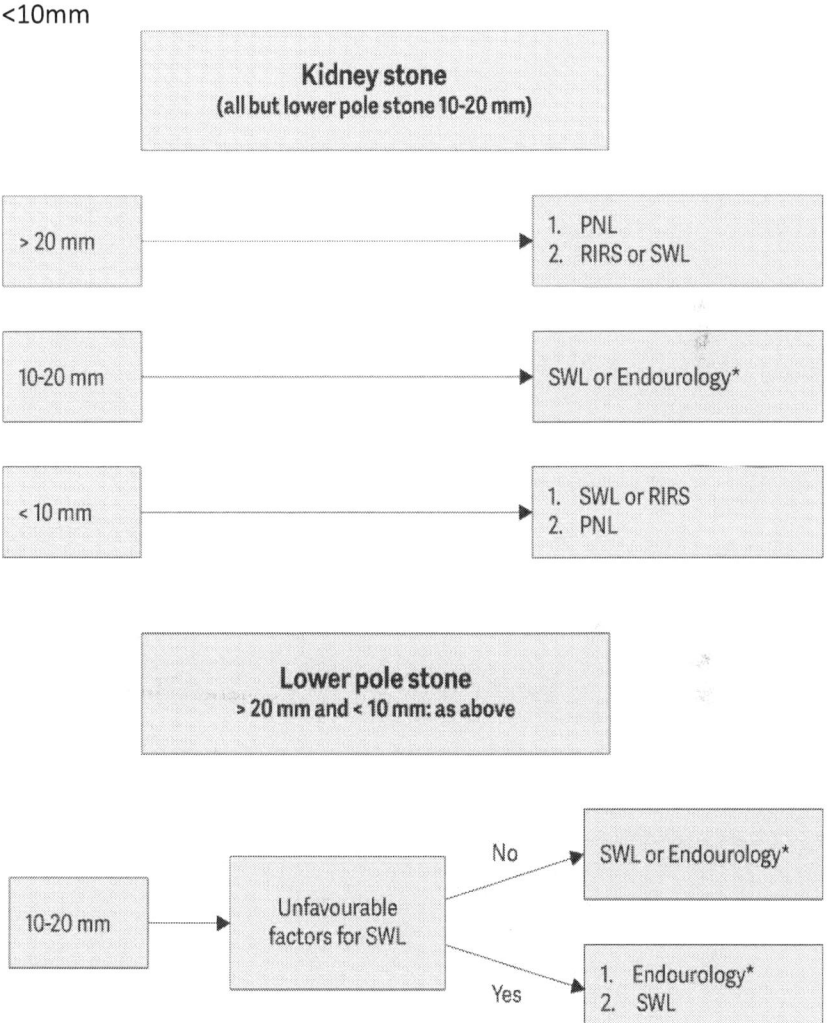

Kidney stone (all but lower pole stone 10-20 mm)

- > 20 mm → 1. PNL 2. RIRS or SWL
- 10-20 mm → SWL or Endourology*
- < 10 mm → 1. SWL or RIRS 2. PNL

Lower pole stone > 20 mm and < 10 mm: as above

- 10-20 mm → Unfavourable factors for SWL
  - No → SWL or Endourology*
  - Yes → 1. Endourology* 2. SWL

Figure (8) EAU guidelines for the management of kidney stones.

Proximal Ureteral Stone

- **> 10 mm** → 1. URS (ante- or retrograde)
  2. SWL
- **< 10 mm** → SWL or URS

Distal Ureteral Stone

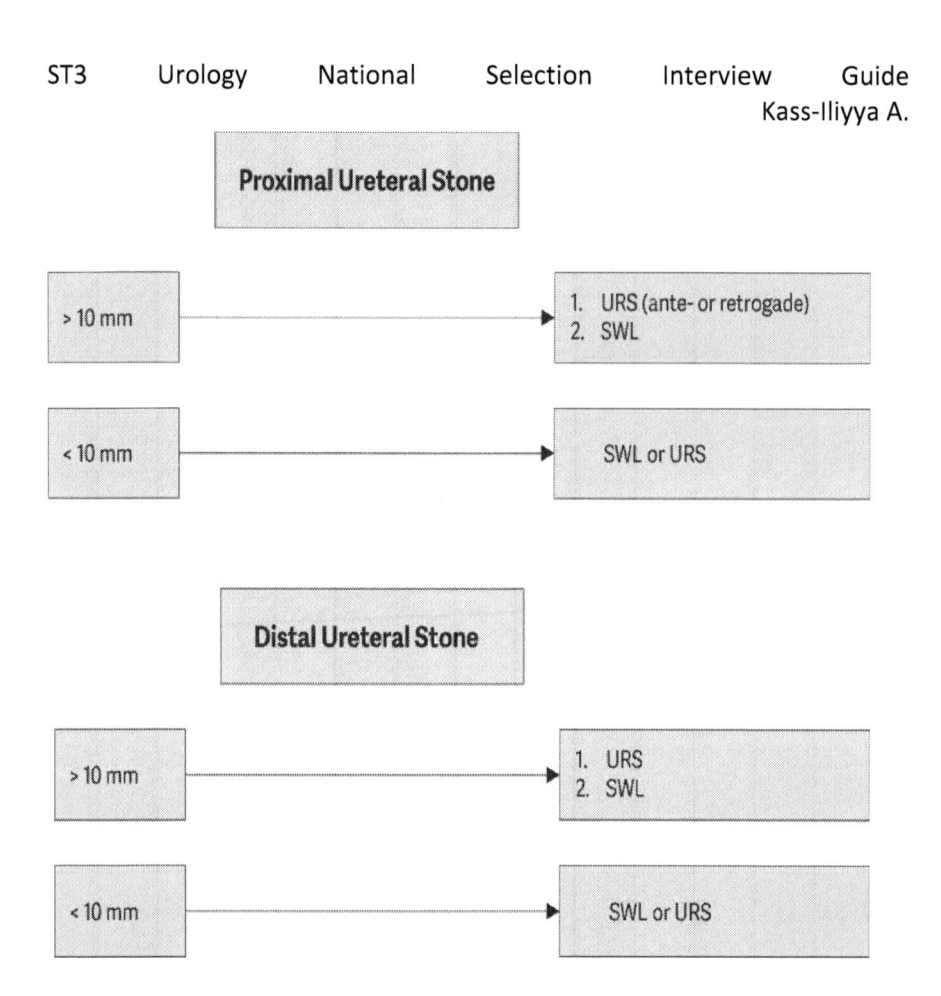

- **> 10 mm** → 1. URS
  2. SWL
- **< 10 mm** → SWL or URS

Figure (9): EAU guidelines for the management of ureteric stones.

4.8. Urinary incontinence

Female stress incontinence (oxford handbook, FRCS viva book)
History taking, examination (cough test, Q-Tip test), clinic based questionnaire (ICS-female Short form) and tests (pad test), other investigations, management (conservative, surgical), types of surgery for SI; synthetic tapes, autologous sling, colposuspension, paravaginal shelf repair, Marshal Marchetti. Different types of tapes; TOT or TVT what is the difference between the two in terms of success rate and complications. Role of urodynamic in investigating incontinence and when to perform.

Here is a summary of the initial assessment of urinary incontinence in general and afterwards I include an assessment of stress urinary incontinence per se:

Evaluation of urinary incontinence
History
It's very important to ask about the following in the history
Type of incontinence (SUI, UUI, MUI)
LUTS (storage or voiding)
Triggers (cough, sneezing, exercise, position, urgency)
Frequency of incontinence episodes
Severity of incontinence (usually assessed with no of pads)
Degree of bother
Bowel function
Sexual dysfunction
POP in women
Validated questionnaire (ICIQ-UI short form)
RED FLAG symptoms
🚩
(PAIN, HAEMATURIA, RECURRENT UTI, VOIDING SYMPTOMS, HX OF PELVIC SURGERY OR RADIOTHERAPY)

Risk factors:
Abdominal/pelvic surgery (RED FLAG)
Rx (RED FLAG)
Neurological disorders
Obsteteric and gynaecology history
Medications (alpha blockers/agonists, diuretics, colchicine, caffeine, sedatives, antidepressants, antipsychotics, and antihistamines)

Physical examination:
Women
Pelvic examination (Supine, Standing, left lateral position w Sim's speculum)
Ask to cough and inspect for
   Anterior and posterior vaginal wall prolapse
   Uterine or vaginal vault descent
   Urinary leakage (stress test)
Internal pelvic examination to assess
   Strenght of pelvic floor muscle
   Bladder neck mobility
Inspect vulva for oestrogen deficiency
Calculate BMI
Both sexes
Examine abdomen (palpable bladder)
Neurological examination (gait, anal reflex, perineal sensation, lower limb funciton)
DRE to exclude
   Constipation
   Rectal mass
   Test anal tone
RED FLAG SIGNS
🚩
(NEW NEUROLOGICAL DEFICIT, HAEMATURIA, URETHRAL, BLADDER OR PELVIC MASSES, AND SUSPECTED FISTULA).
Basic investigations
Bladder diaries
Fluid intake
Frequency and volume of urine voided
Incontinent episodes
Pad usage
Degree of urgency
Urinalysis and culture
Flow rate and post-void residual (PVR) volume
   150 ml for accurate result
   PVR Less than 50 normal more than 200 abnormal, 50-200 requires clinical correlation)
Pad testing
   Performed with a full bladder

Pad weight gain more than 1 g is + for 1h test
Pad weight gain more than 4 g is + for 24h test
Further investigations
Blood tests, imaging (USS) and cystoscopy: indicated for
Complicated cases with persistent or severe symptoms
Haematuria
Bladder pain
Voiding difficulties
Recurrent UTIs
Abnormal neurology
Previous pelvic surgery
Previous Rx
Suspected extra urethral incontinence
Urodynamics
In SUI distinguishes between
Hypermobility ALPP > 90-100 cmH2O
ISD (Intrinsic Sphincter Deficiency) ALPP < 60 cmH2O
Detects DO: contractions during filling or abnormal pressure rise with position change
Detects poor bladder compliance
Ambulatory urodynamics: more physiological
Videourodynamics:
Movement of proximal urethra and bladder neck with filling or provocation, also DSD, VUR)
Sphincter EMG:
provides information on synchronization between the detrusor and EUS.

If the question is asking specifically about stress incontinence, then you might find this summary of assessment useful:
Stress Urinary Incontinence:
50% OF UI in women
Intrinsic loss of urethral strength and/or
Urethral hypermobility
Risk factors for female SUI
Childbirth
Ageing
Oestrogen withdrawal
Previous pelvic surgery
Obesity

Risk factors for male SUI
EUS damage (pelvic *, RP, Pelvic surgery, Rx)
Other risk factors
Neurological disorders (SCI, MS, Spina bifida)
Investigation of SUI
Women
Stress test (cough)
Pad test (no and weight of pads)
Pelvic exam
POP
Elevation of an existing anterior wall prolapse will unmask any occult sphincter incompetence
Oestrogen status

Q-tip test
Lithotomy position
Bladder comfortably full
Well lubricated sterile cotton-tipped applicator inserted into bladder
Applicator withdrawn to point of resistance (bladder neck)
Resting angle from horizontal recorded
Patient asked to strain and the degree of rotation is assessed
> 30 degree resting or straining angle from the horizontal defines hypermobility.
Urethral pressure profile
Urodynamics recommended before surgery for SUI if
Suspicion of DO
Previous surgery for SUI or anterior compartment prolapse
Voiding dysfunction
Men
Abdominal exam (palpable bladder)
External genitalia exam (penile abnormalities)
DRE
Flow Rate and PVR
Upper tract imaging if BOO
Treatment of SUI
Conservative treatment
PFMT (Pelvic Floor Muscle Training)
Eight contractions, three times per day
Improves symptoms in 30% of women with mild SUI

Lifestyle modification
Weight loss
Stop smoking
Avoid constipation
Modify fluid intake
Biofeedback
Info on strength of PF contraction is presented as visual, auditory or tactile signal.
Medication
Duloxetine: inhibits reuptake of both serotonin and noradrenaline increases sphincteric muscle activity during bladder filling.
Extracorporal magnetic innervation
pulsed magnetic field to stimulate the nerves of the sphincter and pelvic floor
High frequency electrical stimulation
No proven benefit in SUI
Surgical Treatment
Urethral bulking agents
Retropubic suspension
Suburethral slings
Artificial urinary sphincters
Injection therapy
Injection bulking material into bladder neck and periurethral muscles
Indication:
Female stress incontinence secondary to ISD with normal bladder function. There is evidence of benefit in urethral hypermobility.
Contraindications
UTI
Untreated OAB
Bladder neck stenosis
Success rates (50-80%). Repeat treatments are often required. Therefore, bulking agents are not commonly used as a first-line intervention.
Complications:
Temporary retention (2-15%)
De novo UI (6-12%)
UTI (5%)
Haematuria (5%)
Distant migration of particles (granuloma formation)
Retropubic suspension

Indication
Urethral hypermobility
Lower chance of benefit in patients with significant ISD.
Types of Surgery
Burch colposuspension
Vagino-obturator shelf/ paravaginal repair
Marshall-Marchetti-Krantz procedure (MMK)
Burch colposuspension: see Figures (10,11)
Most widely used technique
Vaginal wall is elevated and attached to lateral pelvic wall
It is an option for patients with concurrent SUI and anterior vaginal wall prolapse.
Approximating the paravaginal fascia to the iliopectineal ligament of Cooper's. See Figure (10)
Success rates (90%) at 1y and 970%) at 5 y.
Complications
Posterior compartment prolapse (10-25%)
De novo urgency incontinence (15%)
Voiding dysfunction (10%)

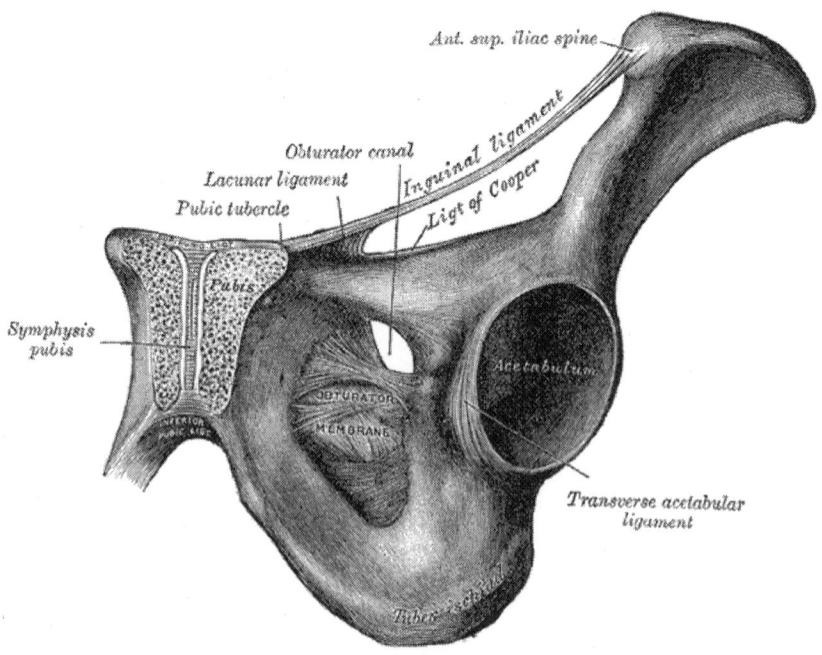

Figure (10) The Iliopectineal ligament of Cooper's

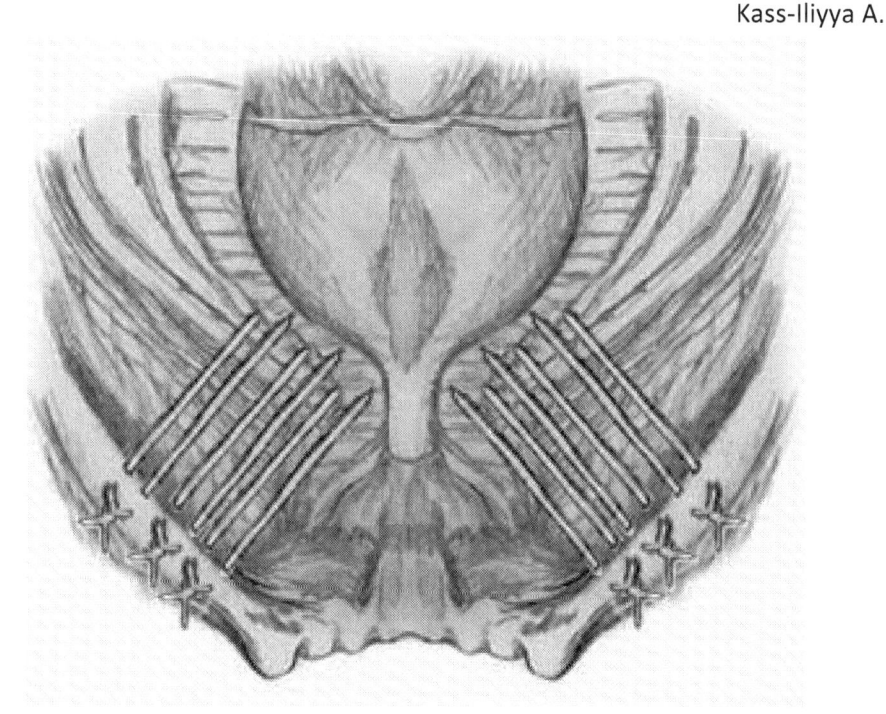

Figure(11) Burch Colposuspension

Vagino-Obturator shelf/paravaginal repair
In some cases, a cystocele develops because the front vaginal wall tears away from its lateral attachment to the pelvic sidewalls, resulting in a paravaginal defect. When this happens, a simple anterior repair is not appropriate, as it won't correct the problem
Variant of the Burch procedure
Sutures from the paravaginal fascia are passed through the obturator fascia to attach to the arcus tendoneus fascia
The aim is to dispense the tension on the paravesical tissues laterally to reduce the risk of prolapse.
Success rate 85%

Marshall-Marchetti-Krantz (MMK) Procedure
Sutures are placed on either side of the urethra at the bladder neck level and tied to the hyaline cartilage of the pubic symphysis.
Short term success 90% (declines over time)
Complications: 3% risk of osteitis pubis. (analgesia, bed rest, steroids)

Suburethral tapes and slings
Types of Sling
Synthetic tapes
monofilamentous polypropylene mesh
Retropubic tape (TVT)
Transobturator tape (TOT)

Autologous
Rectus fascia, fasica lata, vaginal wall
Non-autologous
Fascia lata from cadaveric tissue
Retropubic tapes (TVT):
Midline anterior vaginal incision over the mid-urethra
Trocars inserted either side of the urethra and perforate through the endopelvic fascia into the lower abdominal wall in the midline, just above the pubic bone
Success rates 90% at 1 y 80% at 5 y
TVT vs colposuspension
Ward Hilton studies, similar efficacy at 5y.
TVT have lower OAB symptoms and prolapse (1.8% vs 7.5%)
Transobturator tapes (TOT, TVTO)
Midline anterior vaginal incision over the mid-urethra
Two small incisions lateral to labia majora at level of clitoris
Trocar passed through skin incision, downwards though obturator foramen, exiting alongside urethra on each side (outside to inside)
In TVTO, trocar passes from (inside to outside)
TOT vs TVT:
Similar subjective cure rates at 1 y
TVT better objective cure rates (88% vs 84%)
TOT less voiding dysfunction, blood loss, bladder perforation, shorter operating time
TOT higher vaginal injuries/erosion and pain in the groin/thigh
TVTO vs TVT:
Similar objective cure rates
Increased risk of leg pain
Mini tapes
Self-retaining, inserted via a single vaginal incision
short-term success 80-90%

results may not be sustained over time

General complications of tapes
Voiding dysfunction (retention, de novo bladder overactivity)
Vaginal, urethra, and bladder perforation or erosions
Pain (groin/thigh with TO route)
Damage to bowel or blood vessels (rare)
Pubovaginal (autologous) slings: see Figure (12)
Not commonly used as a first line surgical procedures for SUI
Commonly a segment of rectus fascia (10-20 cm) is harvested and sutured placed on both ends
Sling placed under mid urethra though endopelvic fascia
Suture ends tied
Autologous slings vs colposuspension
Autologous slings have better outcome
Autologous slings have higher complications (UTI, Voiding dysfunction, urge incontinence)

Figure (12) Pubovaginal (autologous) slings

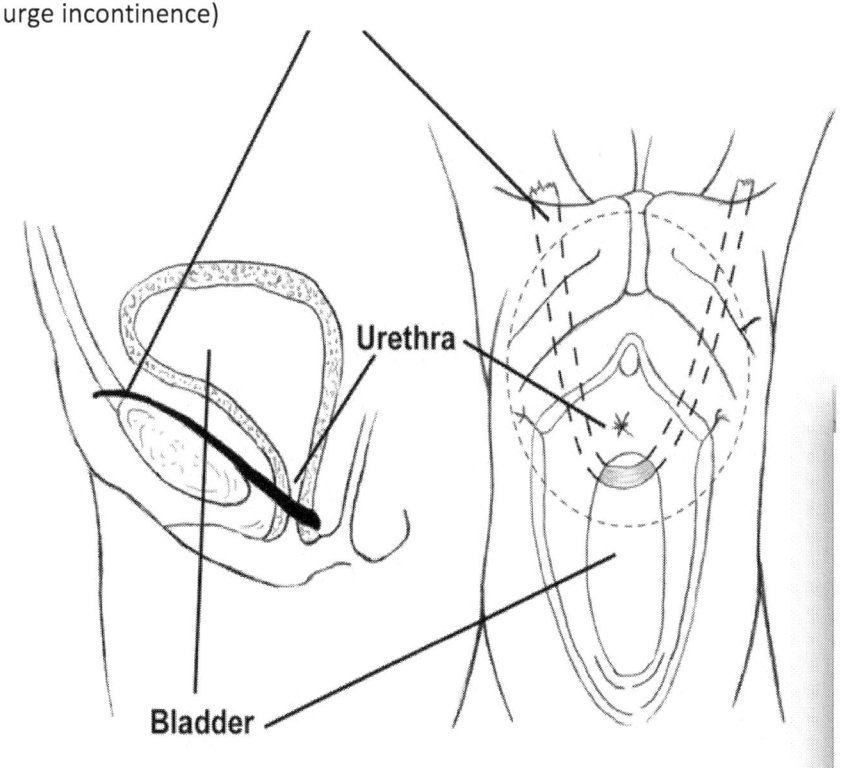

4.9. Haematuria

Haematuria in a male (oxford handbook, FRCS viva book, EAU guidelines)
History:
Visible, non-visible, symptomatic, asymptomatic, Loin pain, dysuria, LUTS (Storage symptoms and bladder pain), Recent upper respiratory tract infection. Recent trauma.
Transient causes: Vigorous exercise, recurrent UTIs, menstruation.
Risk factors for urological cancers
Kidney: Age, race, gender, smoking, obesity, hypertension, family history,
Bladder: occupational exposure, long term catheter, travel, pelvic radiotherapy
Prostate: geography, lifestyle (mobility)
Risk factors for stones
Diet (salt, animal protein, low fluid intake)
UTI
Family history of stone (cystinuria, Renal tubular acidosis)
Always ask about
Bowel function, sexual function, neurological symptoms.
In females ask about periods regular, irregular, intermenstrual bleeding.
Drug history
Discoloration of urine (Rifampicin, doxorubicin, ingestion of beetroot)
Risk of stone (steroids increase absorption of calcium; chemotherapy increases uric acid)
Risk of bladder cancer (phenacetin abuse, cyclophosphamide)
Anticoagulation therapy (warfarin)
Past Medical History
Diabetes, hypertension, Tuberculosis, Atrial fibrillation, coagulation disorders (haemophilia), gout, hyperparathyroidism, sarcoidosis, Inflammatory bowel disease.
Past surgical history
Urological surgery, previous bowel resection.
Examination should include
Abdominal and pelvic exam, Digital rectal examination in men, vaginal examination to rule out vaginal bleeding.
Clinic tests
Record weight, BMI, BP
Send urine for MSC and cytology (sensitivity 49%, specificity 96%)

NMP 22 (nuclear matrix protein 22) sensitivity 70%, specificity 75%
Send bloods for FBC, UEs, coagulation profile, eGFR, ACR, PCR

Organise imaging
USS Kidney ureter bladder, flexible cystoscopy. CTU if no cause is found, retrograde studies
and ureteroscopy if positive cytology despite negative investigations.
More on Haematuria (Investigations)

Urological investigation of haematuria - VH, s-NVH, a-NVH aged >40, persistent (2/3) a-NVH
Urine culture
Urine cytology
Cystoscopy
Renal Ultrasonography
CT Urography

The role of MDCT urography in the investigation of haematuria
Advantages
Single investigation could obviate the need for the traditional '4-test' approach (IVU, renal
USS, F Cystoscopy, urine cytology)
Good sensitivity and high specificity for diagnosing bladder tumours in patients with visible haematuria (93%, 99%)
Equivalent diagnostic accuracy to retrograde uretero-pyelography
65% sensitivity and 98% specificity for the detection of all urological tumours in patients with haematuria and no prior history of urological malignancy

Disadvantages
Higher radiation dose (a 7-film IVU = 5-10mSV, 3-phase MDCTU = 20-25mSV)
It fails to diagnose a significant proportion of urinary neoplasms (sensitivity for upper tract neoplasms 80%, bladder tumours 60%)
High cost

Recommendation: Targeted approach for using CT
Age > 40y
Macroscopic haematuria
Smoking history
Occupational exposure benzenes and aromatic amines

Should cystoscopy be performed in patients with a-NVH?

AUA recommends cystoscopy in all high-risk patients
Smoking history
Occupational exposure to chemicals or dyes (Benzenes or aromatic amines)
Analgesic abuse (phenacetin)
Pelvic irradiation
Cyclophosphamide treatment
In asymptomatic, low risk patients < 40, it may be appropriate to defer cystoscopy, but urine
cytology should be checked. Having said that; flexible cystoscopy should be recommended to such patients and they make a decision based on their interpretation of low risk.
If no cause for haematuria (VH or NVH) is found with cystoscopy and CT urography, is further investigation necessary?
AUA advises repeat urinalysis, urine cytology, and BP measurement at 6,12,24, and 36 months, with repeat imaging and cystoscopy where dipstick or microscopic haematuria persist
There is evidence unless a patient represents with visible haematuria, repeat urologic investigation in those with persistent dipstick or microscopic haematuria will not identify any additional significant urologic pathology.
Repeat urological investigation in persistent NVH is not necessary unless a patient become symptomatic or develops visible haematuria

Nice guidelines on Haematuria referral for suspected bladder cancer:

Bladder cancer
Refer people using a suspected cancer pathway referral (for an appointment within 2 weeks) for bladder cancer if they are:
aged 45 and over and have:
unexplained visible haematuria without urinary tract infection **or**
visible haematuria that persists or recurs after successful treatment of urinary tract infection, **or**
aged 60 and over and have unexplained non-visible haematuria **and** either dysuria or a raised white cell count on a blood test. **[new 2015]**
Consider non-urgent referral for bladder cancer in people aged 60 and over with recurrent or persistent unexplained urinary tract infection. **[new 2015]**

4.10. Erectile Dysfunction

Erectile dysfunction: (unlikely to be asked in the interview but it's better to be prepared) Definition

consistent or recurrent inability to attain and/ or maintain a penile erection sufficient for sexual intercourse

Epidemiology
52 % of men aged 40-70 y (17% mild, 25% moderate, 10% severe)
Increases with age (40% of men in their 80's)

Aetiology
Psychogenic causes
Organic causes

History
Sexual
Onset
Duration
Erections (nocturnal, early morning, spontaneous)
Ability to maintain erections
Loss of libido
Relationship issues (Frequency of intercourse, sexual desire)

Questionnaire
IIEF 5

Medical/ Surgical
Diabetes
Cardiovascular disease (Intermediate/high risk needs treatment before treating ED)
hypertension
Peripheral vascular disease
Endocrine disorders
Neurological disorders
Pelvic and penile surgery
Radiotherapy
Trauma

Psychosocial
Social stresses
Anxiety
Depression

Coping problems
Patient expectations
Relationship details
Drugs
Current medications
ED treatments already tried
Social
Smoking
Alcohol consumption
Examination
Full physical examination
Cardiovascular
Abdomen
Neurological
BP
DRE
Secondary sexual characteristics
External genitalia (phimosis, penile deformities (peyronie's plaques))
Testicles (presence, size, location)
The bulbocavernosus reflex (integrity of S2-4) (glans squeeze —> anal sphincter contraction)
Investigations
Blood tests
Fasting glucose
Serum (free) testosterone (8-11 am)
Fasting lipid profile
SHBG; U&E; LH/FSH; prolactin; PSA; Thyroid function test (selective cases)
Nocturnal penile tumescence and rigidity testing
Rigiscan device
number, duration, rigidity of nocturnal erections
useful for diagnosing psychogenic ED
Penile colour doppler Uss:
Arterial peak systolic and end diastolic velocities pre and post PGE1 injection
Cavernosography:
Measurement of penile blood flow after intracavernosal injection of contrast and artificial erection (to identify venous leaks)
Penile arteriography

Pudendal arteriography before and after erection to identify those needing arterial bypass surgery
MRI
Assess penile fibrosis and severe cases of Peyronie's disease

Treatment of Erectile Dysfunction

Correct reversible causes
Alter lifestyle
Stop smoking
Change medications

Psychosexual therapy
Sex education
Psychosexual counselling
Instruction on improving partner communication skills
Cognitive therapy
Behavioural therapy
Pharmacotherapy

Drug therapy
PDE5 Inhibitors
Types: see Figure (13)
Mechanism of action: see Figure (14)

PDE5I	Doses (mg)	Half-life	Effective within	Duration of action	Common side effects
Sildenafil (Viagra)	25/50/100	3.7h	30–60min	Up to 4–5h	Headache, dizzy, GI upset, flushing, nasal congestion, blurred vision
Vardenafil (Levitra)	5/10/20	3.9h	25–60min	Up to 4–5h	As above
Tadalafil (Cialis)	2.5/5/10/20	17.5h	30min to 2h	Up to 36h	As above

Free NHS prescription (SLS Schedule 11) applies for certain conditions including: diabetes, spinal cord injury, multiple sclerosis, Parkinson's disease, polio, spina bifida, one gene neurological disease, severe pelvic injury, prostate cancer, prostatectomy, radical pelvic surgery, renal failure (treated by dialysis or transplant), for 'severe distress' and patients already receiving NHS ED treatment on 14th September, 1998.

Figure (13) different types of PDE5I, duration of action and common side effects.

Sildenafil (Viagra), tadalafil (Cialis), vardenafil (Levitra)
Enhance cavernosal smooth muscle relaxation
Block the breakdown of cGMP by phosphodiesterase
Success 80%
Early use after RP is recommended

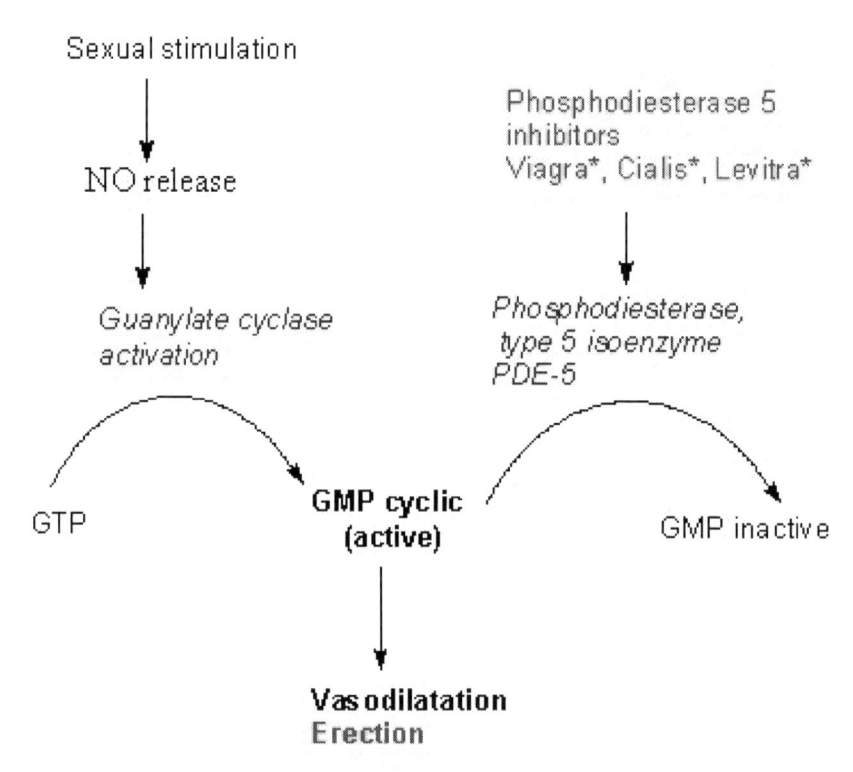

Figure (14) Mechanism of action of PDE5I

Contraindications:
Nitrates
Recent myocardial infarction
Recent stroke
Hypotension
Unstable angina
NAION (Non arteritic anterior ischaemia optic nerve neuropathy)
Cautions

Intermediate/high risk cardiovascular disease (needs cardiac review)
Alpha blockers use
Groups with predisposition to priapism

Dopamine receptor agonist: see Figure (15)

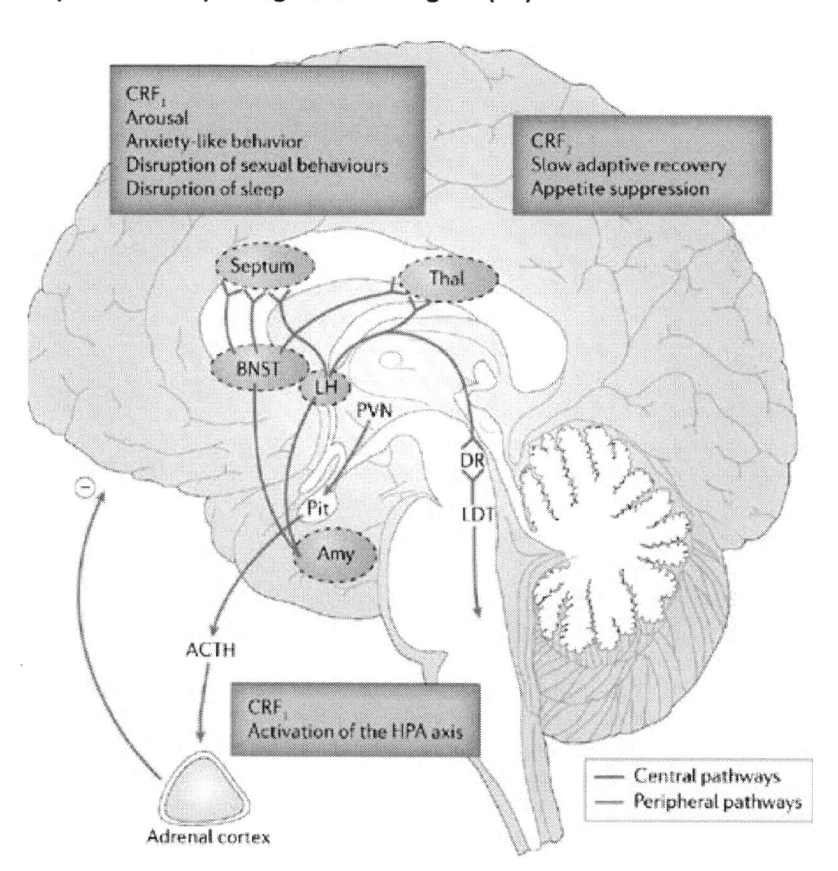

Figure (15) Brain anatomy showing paraventricular nucleus of the hypothalamus (PVN)

Apomorphine: sublingually, acts centrally on dopaminergic receptors in the paraventricular nucleus of the hypothalamus to enhance and coordinate the effect of sexual stimuliciles.

Intraurethral therapy http://www.muserx.com/hcp/local-vasodilation-therapy-for-ed/mechanism-of-action.aspx
Synthetic prostaglandin E1 (PGE1) pellet (Alprostadil) intra urethrally

PGE1 increases cAMP within the corporal smooth muscle, resulting in muscle relaxation.
SEs: Penile and urethral pain, priapism, local reactions.

Intracavernosal injection therapy
Alprostadil (Caverjet ™)
papaverine (PDE inhibitor)
In combination with phentolamine (alpha antagonist) or PGE1

Contraindications:
Sickle cell disease
High risk candidates for priapism

Vacuum erection device
When pharmacotherapies have failed.
Three components:
Vacuum chamber
Pump
Constriction band
Penis is placed in chamber,
Vacuum created increases blood flow to corpora cavernosa,
Constriction band is placed on the base of the penis to maintain rigidity.

Contraindication:
Anticoagulation therapy
Side effects
Penile coldness
Bruising

Microvascular arterial bypass and venous ligation surgery
Increase arterial inflow and decrease venous outflow
Rarely used now.

Penile prosthesis
Semi rigid or Malleable
Inflatable (2 chamber, 3 chamber)

Indications
Other therapies failed
Peyronie's disease
Trauma
penile fibrosis (i.e. secondary to priapism)
High satisfaction rates (90%)

SEs:
Infection

Erosion
Mechanical failure
Penile shortening
Glans may not fully engorge

Testosterone replacement therapy
Indications
Hypogonadism
Oral
Buccal
Intramuscular
Pellet
Transdermal patch
Gel forms
Check: PSA, Hb, LFT, before and after starting treatment

5. The Emergency station

Again this is often predictable as there are limited emergencies in Urology and one should really master these

Example questions

TUR Syndrome
Post TURP Bleeding
Infected obstructed kidney in a diabetic
Acute retention and insertion of suprapubic catheter
Fournier's gangrene (Diabetic, catheterised patient)
Testicular torsion
Renal trauma (Degrees of trauma)

ALL OF THESE SCENARIOS ARE WELL COVERED IN THE FRCS VIVA BOOK.

We would start with ABCDE approach in most of the emergency stations. You wouldn't need
to waste so much time talking about these but here is a comprehensive summary of how to assess each system and how to resuscitate the patient, mostly adopted from the ATLS book in a trauma patient, but the principles are similar.

General approach to an emergency patient
ABCD
Airway
Inspection (foreign bodies, facial, mandibular fractures)
Chin lift or jaw thrust manoeuvre
If patient communicates verbally, airway not likely to be in immediate jeopardy.
If GCS < 8 they need definitive airway

Breathing and ventilation
Chest exposed
Inspect
Auscultate
Palpate

Injuries that can impair ventilation include (This is mainly in trauma, might not apply necessarily in Urological emergencies, but it's worth knowing)
Tension pneumothorax
Flail chest and pulmonary contusion

Massive hemothorax
Open pneumothorax
Circulation with haemorrhage control
Blood volume and cardiac output
Hypotension must be considered hypovolemic in origin until proved otherwise
Clinically: level of consciousness, skin colour, and pulse. (could be assessed within seconds). (Elderly patients have limited physiological reserve and children have abundant reserve)
Level of consciousness:
Blood loss causes impaired cerebral perfusion and results in altered level of consciousness.
Skin colour:
Pink skin in face and extremities rarely has critical hypovolemia.
Ashen, grey facial skin, white extremities.
Pulse
Assess for quality rate and regularity.
Rapid thready pulse, is sign of hypovolemia.
Absent central pulse necessitates immediate resuscitative action
Bleeding
External haemorrhage
Manual pressure on the wound
Pneumatic splinting devices
Tourniquet
Hemostats
Disability
Rapid neurological evaluation
Level of consciousness
Papillary size and reaction, lateralizing sigs, and spinal cord injury
GCS (best motor response)
Exposure
Complete exposure
Warm blankets
External warming device
IV fluids warmed
Warm room temperature

Resuscitation

Airway
Jaw thrust or chin lift
If unconscious and no gag reflex, then oro-pharyngeal airway can help temporarily (Guedel)
Intubation if not maintaining airway.

Breathing/Ventilation/Oxygenation
Intubate if compromised airway due to mechanical factors, ventilatory problems or unconscious.
Surgical airway if intubation not possible
Chest decompression immediately if tension pneumothorax is suspected
Supplemental oxygen
If not intubated should have mask-reservoir device to achieve optimal oxygenation.
Pulse oximeter to monitor saturation

Circulation and bleeding control (This is very important for Urology)
Two large calibre intravenous (IV) catheters should be introduced.
Draw blood for type and cross-match baseline hematologic studies including pregnancy test.
Definitive control of haemorrhage is essential
Operation, angioembolization and pelvic stabilization.
IV fluid with Crystaloids
1-2 litres of isotonic solution to achieve an appropriate response in the adult patient should be warmed. If unresponsive to bolus IV therapy **blood transfusion may be required**. Be aware of hypothermia

Adjuncts to primary survey
ECG
Urinary catheter
Gastric catheter
Ventilatory rate
ABG, Pulse oximetry
Blood pressure
X-ray examination
ECG
Tachycardia, AF, Premature ventricular contraction, ST changes can indicate blunt cardiac injury. PEA can indicate cardiac tamponade, tension pneumothorax, profound hypovolemia. Bradycardia, aberrant conduction and premature beats indicate hypoxia and hypo perfusion.

Urinary catheters
Urine output

Contraindicated in suspected urethral injury (blood at meatus, perineal ecchymosis, blood scrotum, high riding prostate, pelvic fracture), retrograde urethrogram should be done if suspected before insertion of catheter.

Gastric catheters
Reduce stomach distention ad decrease risk of aspiration
Other monitoring
Ventilatory rate and ABG
Adequacy of respiration
Pulse oximetry
Measures the oxygen saturation of haemoglobin, but not the partial pressure of oxygen. Value should be compared with ABG reading.
Blood pressure
X-ray examination and diagnostic studies.
AP chest and pelvic films.
FAST and DPL are useful for detection of occult intra-abdominal blood.
Haemorrhagic shock in injured patient
Is the patient in shock?
Reliance on BP alone may cause delay
Compensatory mechanisms may preclude a measurable fall in systolic bp until up to 30% of the patient's blood volume is lost.
Pulse rate
Respiratory rate
Skin circulation
Pulse pressure
Tachycardia and cutaneous vasoconstriction (typical early physiologic responses to volume loss)
Any injured patient who is cool and has tachycardia is considered to be in shock until proven otherwise
Elderly patients may not exhibit tachycardia
    Limited cardiac response to catecholamine stimulation
    Use of B lockers
    Pacemaker
Normal haematocrit does not exclude significant blood loss
Base deficit and lactate levels are useful to determine presence and severity of shock.
Different causes of the shock state
Haemorrhagic or non-haemorrhagic
Cardiogenic
Cardiac injury, tamponade, air embolus, myocardial infarction.

Investigations: ECG, CK, Echo, FAST.
Signs: tachycardia, muffled heart sounds, and dilated engorged neck veins with hypotension resistant to fluid therapy.

Tension pneumothorax
Mediastinal shift, impaired venous return, fall cardiac output
Signs: Acute respiratory distress, subcutaneous emphysema, absent breath sounds
Hyper-resonance to percussion, tracheal shift

Neurogenic
Intracranial injuries do not cause shock
Signs: hypotension without tachycardia or cutaneous vasoconstriction
Should be treated first as hypovolemic shock, but failure to restore organ perfusion suggests either continuing haemorrhage or neurogenic shock.

Septic shock
Might be confused with hypovolemic shock or both present
Tachycardia, cutaneous vasoconstriction, impaired urinary output, decreased systolic pressure and narrow pulse pressure.

Haemorrhagic shock in injured patients.
Classification of haemorrhage
Class I
Individual who has donated a unit of blood
Class II
uncomplicated haemorrhage, crystalloid fluid resuscitation is required.
Class III
Complicated haemorrhage, at least crystalloid infusion is required and perhaps blood replacement
Class IV
Preterminal event

Class I hemorrhage (15% blood volume loss)
750 ml
PR <100
BP Normal
PP Normal or increased
RR 14-20
UO >30
CNS Slightly anxious
Fluid replacement crystalloid

Class II haemorrhage (15-30% blood loss)
750-1500
PR 100-120

BP Normal
PP Decreased
RR 20-30
UO 20-30
CNS Mildly anxious
Fluid replacement crystalloid
Class III (30-40% blood loss)
1500-2000
PR 120-140
BP Decreased
PP decreased
RR 30-40
UO 5-15
CNS Anxious, confused
Fluid replacement crystalloid and blood +_ surgical intervention

Class IV (>40%)
>2000
PR >140
BP Decreased
PP Decreased
RR > 35
UO Negligible
CNS Confused, lethargic
Fluid replacement, Crystalloid and blood + surgical intervention

Initial management of haemorrhagic shock
What can I do about shock?
Stop bleeding and replace volume loss
ABCDEs
Vital signs, urinary output, and level of consciousness are essential
Airway and breathing
Establish a patent airway with adequate ventilation and oxygenation
Supplementary oxygen is supplied
Circulation – haemorrhage control
Controlling obvious haemorrhage
Obtaining adequate intravenous access
Assessing tissue perfusion
Bleeding from external wounds – direct pressure
Rapid intravenous fluid infusion

Neurological exam
Assess cerebral perfusion
Exposure
Decompression of gastric dilatation
Urinary catheterisation
Vascular access
Two large calibre peripheral intravenous catheters
Fluid warmers and rapid infusion pumps are used in the presence of massive haemorrhage.
Forearms antecubital veins most desirable.
Central venous access (Femoral, jugular, subclavian) if no peripheral access possible.
Blood drawn for type and crossmatch, lab analysis, toxicology, pregnancy.
ABG
Chest x-ray document position of central line.
Initial fluid therapy
Warmed isotonic solutions.
Normal saline, ringer lactate
Alternative is hypertonic saline, although there is no evidence of survival advantage.
Initial warmed fluid bolus is given as rapidly as possible 1-2 litres for adults and 20ml/kg for paediatric patients.
3-1 rule, replace each 1 ml of blood loss with 3 ml of crystalloid fluid.
Monitor patient response
Urinary output
Level of consciousness
Peripheral perfusion
Blood pressure
Aware that fluid resuscitation is not substitute for definitive control of bleeding.
Rapid response
Respond rapidly and remain hemodynamically normal after initial fluid bolus.
Surgical consultation and evaluation are necessary
Transient response
Show deterioration of perfusion indices as the initial fluids are slowed to maintenance levels. Either on-going blood loss or inadequate resuscitation.
Most of these patients lost 20-40% of their blood volume

Continued fluid administration and initiation of blood transfusion is indicated.
Rapid surgical intervention is needed.

Minimal or no response
Immediate, definitive intervention
Remember nonhemorrhagic shock (blunt cardiac injury, cardiac tamponade, tension pneumothorax)
CVP monitoring and cardiac ultrasonography helps differentiate between the various causes of shock

Crossmatched, type-specific and type O blood
Fully cross-matched blood is preferable, however it takes 1 hour
Type specific blood can be provided within 10 minutes
Type O paced cells are used if Type specific blood is not available
Rh negative preferred for females of childbearing age

Warming fluids plasma and crystalloid
Heat crystalloid to 39C before using it.
Warmer or microwave oven (blood products cannot be warmed in microwave oven)

Auto-transfusion
Should be considered for any patient with a major hemothorax

Coagulopathy
PT, PTT, Platelets should be measured in the first hour
Transfusion of platelets, cryoprecipitate and FFP should be guided by coagulation parameters including fibrogen levels
Consideration of early blood component therapy should be given to class IV haemorrhage patients.

Calcium administration
Mostly not needed. Maybe harmful.

Special consideration in the diagnosis and treatment of shock

Equating blood pressure with cardiac output
Unrelated, an increase in peripheral resistance for example with vasopressor therapy with no change in cardiac output results in increased blood pressure but no improvement in tissue perfusion or oxygenation.

Advanced age
Decrease in sympathetic activity, deficit in response to catecholamines
Cardiac compliance decreases
Unable to increase hart rate or efficiency of contraction
Atherosclerosis and occlusive disease makes vital organs sensitive to bp reduction
pre-existing volume depletion (diuretic use, malnutrition)

B-blockers may mask tachycardia
Consider early invasive monitoring
Reduction in pulmonary compliance compounds cellular hypoxia
Glomerular and tubular ageing
Athletes
Blood volume increases 15-20%
Cardiac output six-fold
Stork volume 50%
Resting pulse 50
Remarkable ability to compensate for blood loss
Pregnancy
Physiologic hypervolemia, greater blood loss to manifest perfusion abnormalities.
Medications:
B blockers calcium channel blockers alters hemodynamic response to haemorrhage.
Insulin overdose
Long term diuretic hypokalaemia
NSAIDS Platelet function
Hypothermia
Unresponsive to fluid resuscitation
Coagulopathy
Pacemaker
Unable to respond to blood loss
CVP monitoring is invaluable.

5.1. Anaphylaxis

Scenario: A patient becomes breathless few seconds after IVU injection, how would you manage?

Immediately call the cardiac resuscitation team.
Secure airway and intubate if necessary
Administer 100% oxygen by face mask at a rate of 15 litre/minute.
Insert two large-bore venflons into each antecubital fossa
Give intravenous fluids, Elevate patient's legs
Give adrenaline 0.5mg intramuscular injection (1:1000 = 0.5 ml). Repeated every 5 minutes.
Give intravenous chlorpheniramine 10 mg and intravenous hydrocortisone 200mg.
If no improvement transfer to HDU /ITU

5.2. Testicular torsion

Source: FRCS Viva book.
Know the peak age (12-18-year-old) and (1-year-old) bimodal presentation. know the signs and symptoms of torsion (high riding testicle, horizontal lie, acute hemiscrotum, painful to examine (patient does not allow examination), absent cremasteric reflex, mild erythema of scrotal skin, Prehn's sign: pain is worse on lifting the testicle)

Ask about previous episodes of intermittent pain, any urinary symptoms, sexual activity. The window of opportunity is within the first 6 hours, after that the chances of saving the testicle reduce quickly. Therefore, the management is urgent exploration in theatre, so you need to use your communication skills to open a second theatre for example if theatre is not available immediately or escalate to your consultant if you are struggling to get the patient to theatre immediately. Don't waste time organising an ultrasound scan if you suspect torsion as each second counts and USS cannot exclude torsion, (there might be some blood supply in the testicle despite torsion).

Consent for scrotal exploration
Remember how to consent a patient for testicular torsion (BAUS guidance)
Risks and Complications:

Common (greater than 1 in 10) (>10%)
Fixation of **both** testicles is usually required.
It may be necessary to remove the affected testis if it is too damaged to recover.

Occasional (between 1 in 10 and 1 in 50) (2-10%)
It may be possible to feel the stitch used to fix the testicles through the skin.
Blood collection around the testicles which resolves slowly or needs surgical removal.
Possible infection of the incision or the testis needing further treatment.

Rare (less than 1 in 50) (<2%)
Later shrinkage of the testicle, even if the testis is preserved.
No guarantee of fertility. (Common question in the communication skills station)
Hospital-acquired infection
Colonisation with MRSA (0.9% - 1 in 110).
MRSA bloodstream infection (0.02% - 1 in 5000).
Clostridium difficile bowel infection (0.01% - 1 in10,000).
The rates for hospital-acquired infection may be greater in high-risk patients, for example those patients
with long-term drainage tubes;
who have had their bladder removed due to cancer;
who have had a long stay in hospital; or
who have been admitted to hospital many times.

5.3. Post TURP Bleeding

Post TURP Bleed
Scenario is usually elderly patient with cardiac history, post TURP, hypotensive, tachycardic.
Differential diagnosis:
Post TURP bleed,
Cardiac event
See FRCS viva book
Briefly
ABCD approach.
Airway, Breathing
100% high flow oxygen 15L non-rebreather mask, two large bore cannulas (anti-cubital fossa), send bloods for FBC, UEs, Clotting, Cross match 4 units of blood. ECG
Administer fluids (N.saline, or Hartmans)
Check that catheter is not blocked first and irrigation running. If blocked, try and flush with bladder syringe to get the clots out. Inflate catheter balloon to 50 and Apply traction for 20 minutes with catheter balloon against the prostatic fossa.
Give blood transfusion and correct clotting abnormalities.
If pt haemodynamically unstable, or multiple blood transfusions or persistent clot retention, consider taking back to theatre.
In theatre: bladder washout and diathermy. You could use the cold resectoscope working element to break an organised clot without current. You could use the Elick to evacuate clots. If Elick doesn't work; **Bladder syringe could be very effective in this scenario.** If all those manoeuvres fail, open surgery; pfannenstiel incision and pack the prostatic fossa with gauze for 24-48 hours and re-visit. If this fails, the last resort is super-selective internal iliac artery embolization.

5.4. TUR syndrome

See FRCS Viva book

Patho-physiology

Absorption of large volumes of 1.5% glycine solution, resulting in
Dilutional hyponatraemia (osmotic shift of water from plasma into the brain)
Fluid overload (initially pulmonary oedema and cardiac failure, later, bradycardia and decreased systolic pressure)
Glycine toxicity (flashing lights, prickling sensations and facial warmth, bradycardia due to cardiac toxicity)

Detection:

Usually apparent if the patient is awake ie. Spinal TURP
Hypertension might be the only sign if the procedure is done under GA.
Arrhythmias, hypotension and decreased oxygen saturation are late features
1% ethanol in the irrigant and breathalyser for breath alcohol levels
Weighing machines to operating tables.

Prevention

Reduce resection time to 60 minutes
Avoid aggressive resection near the capsule and finish quickly if capsule is breached
Administer frusemide prophylactically if a prolonged procedure is inevitable.
Use of bipolar or laser resection
Reduce height of irrigation fluid (not proven)

Treatment

Mild cases

Furosemide (40) mg intravenously. An alternative is mannitol.
Control any haemorrhage and finish the Op ASAP
Early input from ITU in all cases of TUR syndrome

Severe cases
Call HDU/ITU team early
Central line and invasive arterial monitoring are usually used
Transfer to ITU when stable
Extreme cases
Intubate and ventilate
Hypertonic saline solution (1mmol/litre per hour is recommended) (beware rapid correction can cause central pontine myelinolysis)

As mentioned in the elective scenario section there is always a communication skills elements to these stations, so in this scenario you might be asked to speak to the family or relatives of a patient with TUR syndrome and you might be asked how serious this condition is? Be careful not to down play the potential life-threatening nature of this syndrome as patients do die in extreme cases!

5.5. Renal Trauma

In this scenario you might get a picture of renal trauma and you will be asked about the degree of injury to the kidney according to AUA classification See below.

You need to know the indications for requesting a spiral CT scan with contrast
Penetrating trauma
Any significant mechanism of injury (fall from a height, rapid deceleration)
Blunt injury + Haemodynamic compromise
Blunt injury + visible haematuria
Blunt injury in children + dipstick or visible haematuria

You need to know the absolute indications for exploring the kidney in trauma
Persistent life-threatening blood loss
Renal pedicle avulsion either demonstrated on imaging or during laparotomy by observing expanding pulsatile retroperitoneal haematoma
Penetrating renal trauma

Grades of Kidney Injury: see Figure (16,17)

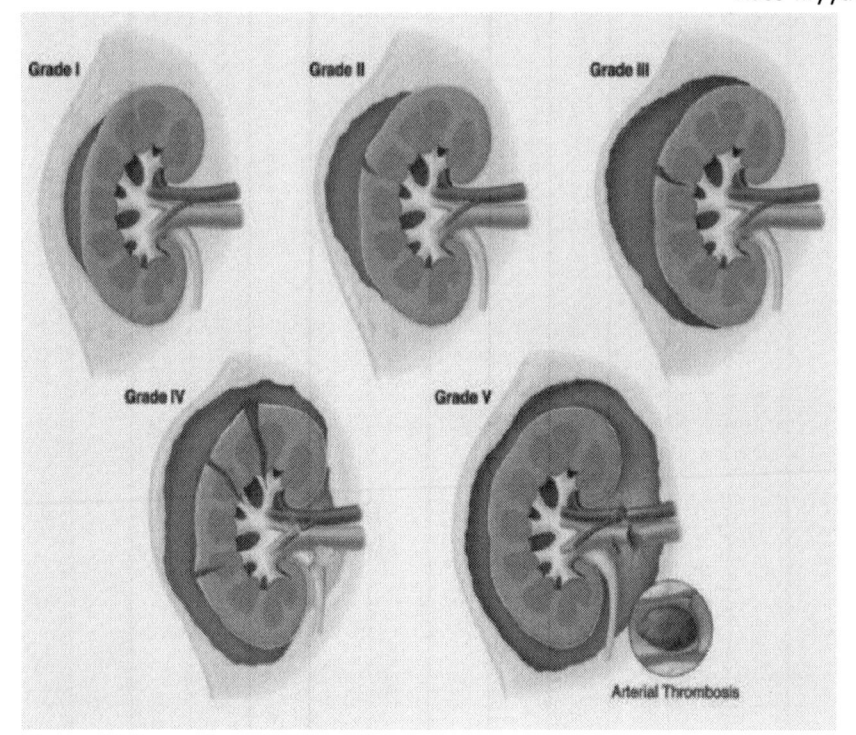

Figure (16): grades of kidney injury.

Table 1: Injury severity scale for the kidney*#	
Grade	Description
1	Contusion or non-expanding subcapsular haematoma, no laceration
2	Non-expanding perirenal haematoma, cortical laceration < 1 cm deep without extravasation
3	Cortical laceration > 1 cm without urinary extravasation
4	Laceration: through corticomedullary junction into collecting system **or** vascular: segmental renal artery or vein injury with contained haematoma
5	Laceration: shattered kidney **or** vascular: renal pedicle injury or avulsion

Figure (17) Grades of renal trauma.

Absolute indications for exploring kidney in trauma:
Presistent life-threatening blood loss that is believed to stem from renal injury
Renal pedicle avulsion (grade V injury) which is suspected clinically, by imaging or by the observation of an expanding pulsatile retroperitoneal haematoma at laparotomy.
Penetrating renal trauma.

5.6. Infected Obstructed Kidney

ST3   Urology   National   Selection   Interview   Guide
Kass-Iliyya A.

You will have an emergency scenario where for example a 73-year-old diabetic lady with previous history of ischaemic heart disease admitted with right loin pain and high temperature 38.5. Bp 95/58, Hr 109. How do you asses and manage?

Standard answer

ABCDE approach

Assess airway.

Administer high flow oxygen 100% 15L via non-rebreather mask

Insert two large-bore cannulas in anti-cubital fossa and take bloods for FBC, UEs, CRP, Clotting, Group and save

Assess GCS

Examine the patient

Obtain an ECG, ABG, Erect Chest x-ray, I catheterise the patient and send urine for M C+S

As the patient is obviously septic (I suspect septic shock, see definitions in page 134) I resuscitate the patient with IV N.saline or Hartman's 1 litre stat if no signs of fluid overload and assess response.

I administer broad spectrum venous antibiotics consulting with microbiology and according to our departmental guidelines. I contact ITU immediately for further help, as this lady is obviously very unwell and might need inotropic support.

I order urgent CT KUB and speak to duty radiologist myself emphasising the urgency of this case and the need to know the underlying diagnosis to start the correct management ASAP. I contact my consultant and keep him/her aware of this case.

If the radiologist tells you to wait until the morning or for another 4 hours. **Refuse** and explain professionally that the CT should "happen now" given the urgency of the situation as this is life threatening. If he refuses again escalate to your consultant immediately.

The CT shows 9mm obstructive stone at the left PUJ how do you manage this patient?

This lady needs urgent drainage of her left kidney, which is the source of her septicaemia.

There are two options:

Insertion of nephrostomy or

Insertion of JJ ureteric stent. (Please see page 98,99 for the pros and cons of each procedure)

You should be able to justify each option. In the UK the common practice in such poorly septic patients who are high anaesthetic risk is to insert a nephrostomy in the first instance. This will better drain the pus, reduce the pressure on the kidney, avoid general anaesthetic and avoid damaging the ureter, however it requires an interventional radiologist and has a small risk of organ injury and bleeding. Two studies addressed the difference between the two procedures in obstructed infected kidneys. Pearle et al and Mokhmalji et al. the first showed no difference the second showed superiority for nephrostomy in terms of success rate of insertion and the speed of controlling the temperature.

5.7. Acute retention of urine

ST3   Urology   National   Selection   Interview   Guide
Kass-Iliyya A.

A 76-year-old man presents to A/E with a painfully distended bladder and an inability to pass urine. How would you manage this patient?
Take a focused **history** (Prior LUTS, duration, severity, any red flags; visible haematuria, recurrent UTIs, any medications Tamsulosin, Finasteride, Anticholinergics, anti-psychotics, strong analgesics, bowel habits and any recent constipation, any neurological deficit or signs of cord compression, recent pelvic surgery, any previous urethral instrumentation)
Examine the patient (including abdomen, testicles, DRE)
Insert a urinary **catheter** (it's very important to record the volume drained)
Urinalysis
FBC, UEs (if chronic retention is suspected)
USS KUB (if chronic retention is suspected, i.e. residual volume >1litre and palpable percussable bladder)

If Creatinine is 450 and USS KUB showed bilateral hydronephrosis, how do you manage?
I would admit the patient
Hourly HR, BP, **Urine output**
If pt produces > 200 ml of urine per hour for 2 consecutive hours I would give replacement N.saline equivalent to 90% of the patient's previous hour's urine output (some replace only 50%)
Daily weight
Daily UEs

What is the mechanism of post-obstructive diuresis?
Physiological and pathological
Physiological: accumulation of fluid, electrolytes and waste products during the preceding period of renal failure.
Pathological: (tubular dysfunction and inappropriate salt and water handling by the kidney)
Defective generation of medullary solute gradient secondary to
Decreased re-absorption of NaCl by the thick ascending limb of the loop of Henle.
Decreased re-absorption of urea by the collecting tubule
Inability to maintain medullary solute gradient secondary to
Increased medullary blood flow (solute washout)
Increased endogenous production of ANP
Poor response of collecting duct to ADH.

What is your definitive management of the patient?
This represent HPR and needs TURP after at least 2 weeks of catheterisation

5.8. Fournier's gangrene

82-year-old diabetic man with long term catheter was admitted with scrotal swelling on examination he has a black skin area on his scrotum.

What is your main diagnosis?

Fournier's gangrene: a form of necrotising fasciitis, affecting the perineum and male genitalia.

Risk factors

Recent instrumentation of the urinary tract
Urethral stricture disease
Local trauma
Paraphimosis
Peri-urethral extravasation of urine
Peri-rectal or peri-anal infections
Recent surgery in the ano-genital area (circumcision or hernia repair)
Presence of long-term catheter
Reduced mobility
Incontinent patient
Immunosuppressed patients (diabetes, alcohol abuse)

How do you assess and manage?

Resuscitate the patient aggressively.

Examination:

Evaluate the perineum, the peri-anal region and the genitals, looking for any areas of skin necrosis and the presence or absence of crepitus of the anterior abdominal wall.

Peri-anal involvement signifies an ano-rectal source, and the presence of skip lesions suggests more extensive involvement.

Prompt diagnosis is critical; usually marked systemic toxicity that is out of proportion to the local finding

Transfer the patient urgently to a urological ward or ITU/HDU depending on the severity of the condition.

Start IVT and IV antibiotics and prepare for surgical debridement

Send bloods (FBC, UEs, LFTs, G&S, and glucose)
Do ABG
Send blood and urine cultures and any obvious pus from the region.
If possible CT scan is useful pre-operatively to identify the possible, source of infection.

What is the most common organism?

A mixture usually.

E-coli is the most common organism this could be combined with Klebsiella, enterococci or anaerobes (bacteroides, fusobacterium, clostridium)

I would administer the appropriate antibiotics after discussion with the microbiologist. Usually triple therapy such as **1) gentamicin, 2) metronidazole and 3) either Augmentin or third generation cephalosporin**

How do you position the patient in theatre? And how extensive your debridement is going to be?

Lithotomy position is the preferred position as it gives you very good exposure to the perineal area.

I will debride all the unhealthy and necrotic tissue until I encounter fresh bleeding from the subcutaneous tissue at the cutting edge.

Are you aware of any techniques to speed up wound healing postoperatively?

Hyperbaric oxygen

Vacuum Assisted Closure (VAC)

6. Communication Skills

This is a very important station and we all tend to somewhat neglect this station as we think it will come to us naturally at the interview. This is a big mistake. **This station needs practice the most! I would recommend spending 15-20 minutes each day for three months practicing this station.**

This station is worth 40 marks which is more than all the other stations except the portfolio station. This highlights its importance. You will usually be given a scenario and an actor will be pretending to be a patient or a relative. He might ask tricky questions or become angry so you need to be skilful at diffusing his anger and addressing his concerns which you might need to explore more often than not.

The bottom line of a good communication with an angry/upset patient is:
Exploring patient knowledge and expectations.
Listening.
Staying calm/handling emotions.
Being very sensitive to patient feeling and breaking information very gradually and in a gentle manner.
Apologising and admitting mistake if there has been one.
Taking responsibility.
Taking action and feeding back/showing that you are serious about the mistake.
Addressing any hidden concerns or undisclosed emotions.
Keeping the patient updated.
Giving the patient means of contact. Every single point of the above carries marks and it is very important to follow these general steps in approaching this station.
Introduce yourself:
Good afternoon, my name is Mr xxx xxxx I am one of the urology registrars working here, I believe it's Mr Smith?
I am here to talk to you about xxxxx.
Set the scene:

Ask if the patient wants anybody else to be present in the room, and explain that you have put your bleep with your colleague so that you won't be interrupted.

Ask the patient/relative what they know so far about the case and explore their expectations: this helps you find out what the patients know so far and what are the areas that you need to focus on. It also buys you some time to prepare what you are going to say next.

Gradually break the news or communicate the task that is required of you: you need to be very careful here not to sound so abrupt as this might show lack of compassion or might upset your patient which you should avoid at all costs. You could be communicating a mistake or bad news

For example: if it's bad news, you could say, "I'm afraid I don't have good news for you today". If it's a mistake you could say, "I'm afraid the operation did not go completely as we would have liked".

Apologise: This is extremely important; it makes a lot of difference to an angry patient and often **scores you lots of points**. You need to apologise and take responsibility. This will help diffuse a heated argument with an angry patient and will show that you are compassionate. That's what most patients are looking for "a recognition of the hurt or damage that a mistake, an error or a complication has caused them". This goes a long way. Even if it wasn't your fault you need to apologise for it as you are part of the team that made the mistake and it's very professional of you to take ownership. You could say something along the lines of "I apologise on behalf of the team".

Don't be defensive: we all tend to be defensive when faced with an accusing angry patient. As doctors we take a lot of pride in our professionalism and integrity and when this is attacked we feel a deep sense of unfairness and occasionally we fall for the knee-jerk reaction of becoming defensive or dismissive. This shows lack of insight, at the end of the day the patient has met you for only few minutes and his judgment is based purely on anger and frustration rather than on facts. There is often nothing personal. You need to be very patient, calm and understanding, and you need to show the patient that you are here to help and that you are on his/her side. You could mention something along the lines of "I am very sorry that you feel that way, I would have probably felt the same, but I am here to help you and I would like to explore your concerns and worries and help you solve them". Show the patient that you are on his side. An example of how not to do it is this response to an angry patient whose elderly mother had a bladder perforation during TURBT. "Well! I'm not sure why you're so angry, as I said before, bladder perforation is a well-known complication of TURBT, it's not our fault, your mum was made aware of this and she accepted the risk and signed the consent form, she's an elderly lady and her bladder wall is very thin so it's no surprise that this has happened, the surgeon didn't do it deliberately, did he?" although this statement might hold a lot of truth it comes across as very defensive, rude and careless and it will certainly guarantee turning the relative from an angry to a furious one. Also in this scenario if the actor is asking whether there has been a mistake, and if you were not involved in the operation yourself, you then really don't know, so all you could say is that "a mistake is possible and I sincerely apologise if this is the case, I will need to speak to the surgeon who performed the operation to find out what exactly happened and get back to you". Having said that, if a mistake was made we will investigate it thoroughly and hold the person responsible accountable. "I just want to make you aware that we do take mistakes in our trust very seriously and we do everything in our power to find the **root cause** (this is a buzz word) and ensure that they do not happen again."

Acknowledge patients' emotions and address them: "You look angry". "You look concerned". Again, this shows that you are observant and sensitive and gives the patient a chance to vent and express his/her feeling which is always a result of a good communication. This will also comfort the patient and make him/her feel better.

Explore patients concerns: This is where some candidates excel in comparison with others. Every actor has hidden concerns that are not so obvious on the surface. For example, a father who had an only son who had an orchidectomy after a missed testicular torsion might be concerned that his son's fertility is affected and therefore he couldn't have the grandchildren that he was longing for. A son whose mother is too ill because of operative complication might be the only carer for his wife and cannot spend too much time with his mother due to his own commitments. Often actors drop clues about their inner concerns without saying them very clearly and the reason for that is that they are testing your listening skills and ability to pick up on those clues and address them as well as addressing the obvious problem. Remember: "**actors don't say things just for the sake of it**". They are all taught to say certain things and if you think that an actor mentioned something that is not related to the problem that you are discussing, **don't brush it off** and move on. If you do, the actor will think that you don't care and that you lack insight! Needless to say, you will lose marks.

Address those concerns one by one. You need to give the patient a realistic picture of how you are going to address their concern. You need to be pro-active. For example when you are communicating with a father whose son had an orchidectomy for a missed torsion that was mistaken for epididmo-orchitis by an A/E doctor 24 hours earlier, you need to apologise for the mistake, investigate who was the responsible doctor in A/E, speak to the doctor, get their views, speak to your consultant and promise to raise this in a **meeting where you discuss policies and procedures** (governance meeting; the patient will not understand what a governance meeting is). It helps to say something along the lines of "I am very sorry about your son, we take mistakes like these very seriously (the word seriously here gives the impression that you are serious about solving this problem and gives the patient some reassurance that you are dealing with this issue appropriately) in our trust and we will do everything we can to make sure that **this will never happen again."**

Give the patient a realistic timeline as to when you are going to get back to them with the outcome.

Give your contact details and the contact details of the urology nurse specialist, consultant secretaries and any relevant healthcare professionals that the patient could contact if they have any worries or concerns.

Ask if they have any other questions or concerns. For example, you could say something like: "Is there **something** else you would like to discuss?" (The word something sounds better in this context than the word anything, it sounds more caring and specific)

If needed, advise the patient that if he is not satisfied with the outcome of the investigation he could raise a complaint, direct him to the complaint department, or PALS (Patient advice and liaison services) where he could be given further advice on how to make a complaint. If he's not satisfied with the hospital response after a complaint, advise him that he could contact the local ombudsman.

General points to remember:
Maintain eye contact.
Respect the patient and never become defensive or condescending.
Listen to the patient.
Apologise when needed and always admit a mistake.
Don't say anything that you are not sure about, don't make false statements to cover up an area which you lack knowledge in. If you don't know the answer to something say: "I am sorry, I am afraid I don't know the answer to this, I will have to investigate and get back to you if that's

OK?" Always arrange a call-back time to show that you are serious about this. (For example, a father asks you: "Is an orchidectomy after a missed torsion going to affect my son's fertility?" The right answer is: "The chances are that his fertility will be preserved but I am afraid that there is no guarantee of fertility". Some candidates might be falsely reassuring and say: "Rest assured your son's fertility will be 100% preserved and removing one testicle is not going to affect his fertility whatsoever as the other testicle will do the job". Although the chances of that are true you can't be 100% sure as the patient might have problems with the other testicle and might have problems with fertility in the future. Another example, you are told that an ST5 was performing a nephrectomy and the operation was complicated by a bowel injury. When you explain this to the patient's relative you could inadvertently say: "The operation was performed by a junior doctor!". Although strictly speaking this is true, it gives the impression that the doctor is ill-experienced and therefore he should not be allowed to operate. However, a good communicator will say something along the lines of, "The operation was performed by a senior trainee who is properly trained and heavily supervised by a consultant".

Be careful how you come across, always put yourself in the patient/relative's shoes and be gentle with your delivery to avoid major upsets.

Communication also features in the other stations which highlights its importance in scoring high in this interview.

For example

Talking to relatives about a patient who was admitted to ITU with severe TUR syndrome.

Talking to a concerned relative about his elderly mother who had staghorn calculi and enquiring about PCNL and what the pre-assessment process entails. (You need to explain in layman terms the C-PEX procedures).

As your patient is in the anaesthetic room you noticed that the anaesthetist is drunk, what would you do? (or your consultant is drunk).

You are contacted by a concerned relative whose father had a CT scan 2 days ago which showed TCC and the relative wants to know what it showed?

Example communication skills scenarios

Remember, whatever the scenario is, if you follow the steps outlined above you will score high in this station.

Talking to an angry relative after an operative complication. (Bladder perforation, bleeding post-nephrectomy, ITU admission etc...).

Talking to an angry relative after a missed diagnosis and serious consequences. Examples include, missed torsion, missed ureteric stone and subsequent admission with life threatening obstructed infected kidney or missed appendicitis (diagnosed as pyelonephritis, patient re-admitted later with perforated appendix and had bowel resection).

Talking to an angry relative after patient discharged from urology with pain and with no diagnosis after normal scans.

Talking to an angry patient whose biopsies went missing and he is very anxious about the results.

Talking to an angry patient who didn't have the desired effect after his operation (worsening LUTS after TURP, still incontinent after a sling).

Talking to a patient who was informed late of an incidental cancer diagnosis. (For example after TURP).

7. The practical skills station

In this station, you will be tested to perform a common urological procedure and will most likely be asked a few questions about it.
The golden rule:
<u>Time is the essence here</u>! Don't waste too much time talking about what you are going to do rather than doing it. This was my fault in my last interview and I was penalised heavily for it. The focus of this station will be mainly on the technical aspect rather than the knowledge aspect. (Of course, you need to have a basic level of knowledge like knowing the name of the instruments). Remember you only have 12 minutes to finish this station. Most stations involve performing a task and then answering questions about it, for example a consent form.
Examples: (Remember this is set at ST3 level competencies, so it is somewhat predictable):
Insertion of suprapubic catheter.
Flexible cystoscopy and TURBT consenting.
Ureteric stenting.
Circumcision.
Suturing and knot tying.

Ureteric stent insertion

You need to know how to assemble a cystoscope:
The parts of the cystoscope are (very important): see Figure (18)
Scope (lens).
Bridge (helps attach the scope to the sheath).
Sheath.
Albarran bridge (attaches directly to the sheath without the need for a bridge).
Visual Obturator (attaches directly to the sheath without the need for a bridge).
Blind Obturator (attaches directly to the sheath without the need for a bridge).
Camera.
Light cable and light source.
Normal Saline for stent insertion.

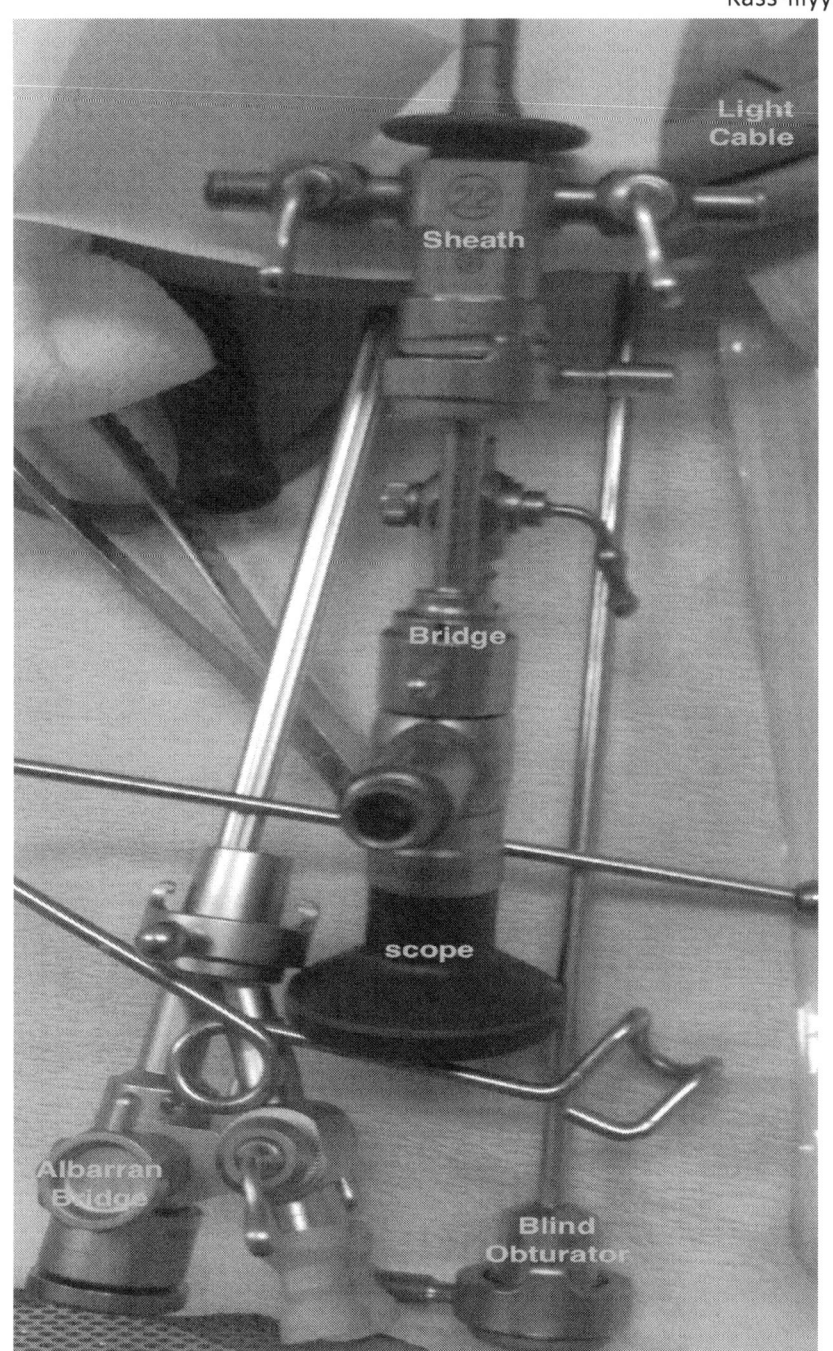

Figure (18) Different parts of the cystoscope

It is safer to use a visual obturator in a male and a blind obturator in a female when first inserting the cystoscope to avoid damaging the urethra. Once you have done the cystoscopy quickly, you need to disconnect the scope, remove the bridge and attach the Albarran bridge instead (called a catheter slide in some hospitals).

Through the Albarran bridge you need to insert a ureteric catheter. You could also load the ureteric catheter with a sensor or PTFE guidewire if the ureteric orifice is small or difficult to access directly with a ureteric catheter. Subsequently you inject a contrast urografin (beware allergy to iodine) 20/20 or 50/50 to perform retrograde uretero-pyelogram to visualise the ureter and the pelvis and then afterward, you insert the guidewire with the floppy end first with fluoroscopy in theatre and once you are satisfied that the guidewire position is in the renal pelvis, you remove the ureteric catheter and keep the wire in place. Next you insert the stent over the guidewire using the pusher to position the upper coil of the stent in the renal pelvis (you will usually see the black mark close to the distal end of the stent), then you withdraw the guidewire to allow the stent to coil in the renal pelvis and the bladder under fluoroscopy guidance. Remember always insert the tapered end of the stent first and the black mark towards the end. (Easy to remember).

Remember the following:

WHO Checklist before stent insertion.

Team introduction, check correct patient, consent form, site of surgery, check side is marked, check patient allergies, any artificial metal work or pacemaker, **if lady in a reproductive age always check for pregnancy because you will need to use fluoroscopy in theatre**, ASA grade, antibiotics administration on induction, VTE prophylaxis, explore any specific concerns.

You might be asked about the different types of stents and guidewires.

Stents

Polymers stents; most commonly used (polyurethane, styrene-ethylene-butylene (C-flex, percuflex)) last 6 months.

Silicone stents (stiffer can last for 1 year).

Metallic stents; for malignant ureteric strictures (Memokath).

Guidewires:

PTFE

Hydrophilic (Terumo)

Hydrophilic tip (Sensor)

Stiff wires (Amplatz Super Stiff)

Insertion of suprapubic catheter

Contraindications:
Suprapubic catheterization is absolutely contraindicated in the absence of an easily palpable or ultrasonographical localized distended urinary bladder.

Suprapubic catheterization is relatively contraindicated in the following situations:

Coagulopathy or patient on anti-coagulants (until the abnormality is corrected).

Prior lower abdominal or pelvic surgery (potential bowel adherence to the bladder or anterior abdominal wall; may recommend that a urologist perform an open cystostomy).

Pelvic cancer with or without pelvic radiation (increased risk of adhesions).

Haematuria due to the risk of seeding of bladder cancer.

Known bladder cancer.

Pelvic fractures (risk of catheter entering a large pelvic haematoma rendering it infected).

Abdominal wall sepsis.

Subcutaneous vascular graft in the suprapubic region (femoro-femoral cross-over graft.).

A common scenario is inserting a suprapubic catheter in a patient with an INR of 2 on warfarin.

It's not safe. You need to reverse the warfarin, and you could consult with haematology or medics on how best to reverse it (beware of patients with metallic heart valve where reversal could lead to valve thrombosis, here you need cardiology/haematology advice, most likely modifying with heparin bridging therapy).

Slow reversal: Vitamin K is an option but takes 4-6 hours to reverse the warfarin, you could use a green venflon to temporarily aspirate some urine if the patient is in agony and cannot wait all that time.

Quick reversal: Beriplex (prothrombin complex concentrate) (30 units/kg) + vitamin K (5mg IV) is the option of choice for a quick reversal; FFP (Fresh Frozen Plasma) is no longer recommended.

Suprapubic catheter side-effects (BAUS consent form) Most procedures have possible side-effects. But, although the complications listed below are well-recognised, most patients do not suffer any problems.

Common (greater than 1 in 10) (>10%)
Temporary **mild burning or bleeding** during urination.

Occasional (between 1 in 10 and 1 in 50) (2-10%)
Infection of the bladder needing antibiotics (occasionally, recurrent infections).
Blocking of the catheter needing unblocking.
Bladder **discomfort** and pain.
Persistent leakage from the water pipe (urethra) which may need a further operation to close the bladder neck.
Development of **stones and debris** in the bladder, causing catheter blockage, and requiring removal or crushing by a further procedure.
Rare (less than 1 in 50) (<2%)
Bleeding requiring irrigation, or additional catheterisation, to remove blood clot.
Rarely, **damage to surrounding structures**, such as bowel or blood vessels with serious consequences, possibly needing additional surgery.

Hospital-acquired infection
Colonisation with MRSA (0.9% - 1 in 110).
MRSA bloodstream infection (0.02% - 1 in 5000).
Clostridium difficile bowel infection (0.01% - 1 in 10,000).

Flexible cystoscopy

The diameter of the flexible cystoscope ranges from 15 to 18 French.
Contraindicated with febrile patients, active UTI.
Usually the scenario entails performing a flexible cystoscopy on a model.
You need to be quick and methodical.
Do the checks.
Correct patient.
Check allergies including LATEX.
Check that the patient doesn't have any of the following:
An artificial heart valve.
A coronary artery stent.
A heart pacemaker or defibrillator.
An artificial joint.
An artificial blood- vessel graft.
A neurosurgical shunt.
Any other implanted foreign body.
A regular prescription for a blood thinning agent such as warfarin, aspirin, clopidogrel (Plavix®), rivaroxaban, prasugrel or dabigatran.
A previous or current MRSA infection.
A high risk of variant-CJD (if you have had a corneal transplant, a neurosurgical dural transplant or injections of human-derived growth hormone).
Ask the patient to empty the bladder and undress.
If patient has artificial sphincter, de-activate it first.
Drape patient from waist down.
Clean with Sterile N.saline.
Insert **Instillagel**:
> Active ingredients of Instillagel are (in each 100 grams):
> Lidocaine Hydrochloride (Local anaesthetic) 2 g (i.e. 2%)
> Chlorhexidine Gluconate Solution (Antiseptic) 0.25 g
> Methyl Hydroxybenzoate (E218) (Antiseptic) 0.06 g
> Propyl Hydroxybenzoate (E216) (Antiseptic) 0.025 g

Explain the procedure to the patient very quickly. Mention the different parts of the urethra as you insert the scope maintaining the lumen in the centre of vision and filling the bladder with irrigation fluid: penile urethra, bulbar urethra, membranous urethra, mention the external sphincter here, the prostatic urethra, mention the verumontanum here, bladder neck, trigone, ureteric orifices, dome, side-walls, anterior wall, and don't forget to perform the J- manoeuvre as well at the end. Then the examiners might ask you about bladder tumours and TURBT consent form.

Withdraw the scope inspecting the urethra carefully, pull the foreskin back if retracted to avoid paraphymosis.

Ask the patient to empty the bladder.

Remember, the information that the flexi can give you about a bladder tumour include:

Size

Location

Solid or papillary

Single or multifocal

Flexible cystoscopy side-effects:

Common (greater than 1 in 10)

Mild burning or bleeding on passing urine for a short period after the operation.

Occasional (between 1 in 10 and 1 in 50)

Infection of the bladder requiring antibiotics.

Rare (less than 1 in 50)

Temporary insertion of a catheter.

Delayed bleeding requiring removal of clots or further surgery.

Injury to the urethra causing delayed scar formation.

Hospital acquired infection

Colonisation with MRSA (0.9% -1 in 110).

Clostridium difficile bowel infection (0.01% -1 in 10,000).

MRSA bloodstream infection (0.02% - 1 in 5000).

Q: On Flexible cystoscopy you find papillary TCC, you book the patient for TURBT, explain the consent form and side effects?

TURBT Side effects (BAUS Consent form)

Common (greater than 1 in 10)

Mild burning or bleeding on passing urine for short period after operation.

Need for additional treatments to the bladder to prevent later recurrence of tumours.

Occasional (between 1 in 10 and 1 in 50)

Infection of the bladder needing antibiotics.

No guarantee of cancer cure by this operation alone.

Recurrence of the bladder tumour and/or incomplete removal.

Rare (less than 1 in 50)

Delayed bleeding needing removal of clots or further surgery.

Damage to drainage tubes from kidney (ureters) needing additional therapy.
Injury to the urethra causing delayed scar formation.
Perforation of the bladder **(Important! (2%) interview question)** needing a temporary urinary catheter or open surgical repair. (You could mention here the 'obturator kick' as a risk factor for lateral tumours)

Hospital acquired infection
Colonisation with MRSA (0.9% -1 in 110).
MRSA bloodstream infection (0.02% -1 in 5000).
Clostridium difficile bowel infection (0.01% -1 in 10,000)
If you were asked how do you avoid the Obturator kick you could answer as follows
Reduce the current (you might need to use coagulation instead of cutting)
Paralyse the patient (General anaesthesia with muscle relaxant) to minimize thigh adduction
Obturator nerve blockade
Use of laser resectors
Also some surgeons advise to empty the bladder to increase the thickness of the muscle layer and cause less nerve irritation. (It becomes thin if the bladder is stretched too much)

Circumcision

Kit
Marking pen
Scalpel/ Blade Size 10 (the bigger the size the smaller the blade)
Mosquito Hemostats/forceps (2 straight artery forceps and one curved artery forcep)
Scissors
Probe to release adhesions if present
Bipolar diathermy
Adson Tissue forceps
Sutures
Needle holder
3-0 Vicryl rapid for skin
Local anaesthetic (for example 0.5% bupivacaine 10 ml)

Techniques of circumcision
Dorsal slit
Shield and clamp (using devices)
Mogen clamp. See Figure (19)
Plastibell. See Figure (20)
Excision
Sleeve technique

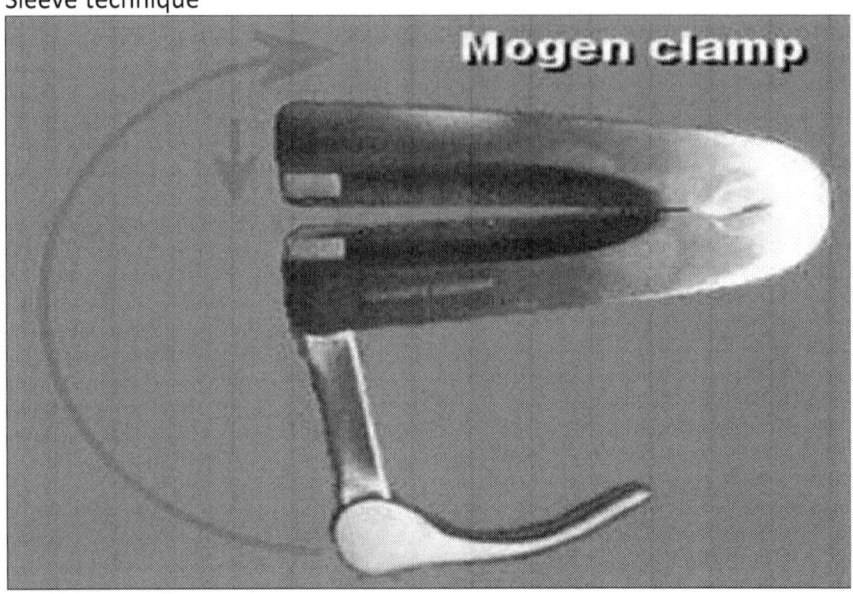

Figure (19) The Mogen clamp (device circumcision)

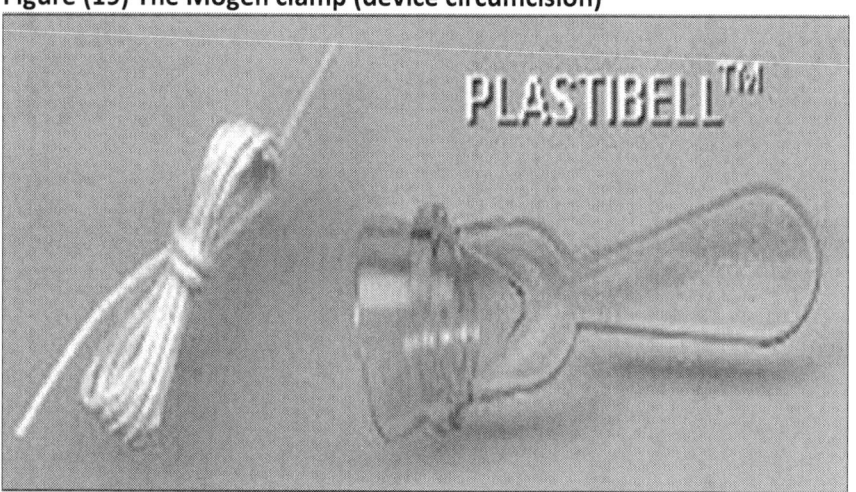

Figure (20) Plastibell device for circumcision

Consent form for circumcision:
Common (greater than 1 in 10)
Swelling of the penis lasting several days.
Occasional (between 1 in 10 and 1 in 50)
Bleeding of the wound occasionally needing a further procedure.
Infection of the incision requiring further treatment and/or casualty visit.
Permanent altered or reduced sensation in the head of the penis.
Persistence of the absorbable stitches after three to four weeks, requiring removal.
Rare (less than 1 in 50)
Scar tenderness.
Failure to be completely satisfied with the cosmetic result.
Occasional need for removal of excessive skin at a later date.
Permission for biopsy of abnormal area on the head of the penis if malignancy is a concern.
Hospital -acquired infection
Colonisation with MRSA (0.9% -1 in 110).
Clostridium difficile bowel infection (0.01% -1 in 10,000).
MRSA bloodstream infection (0.02% -1 in 5000)

IV Contrast with renal impairment and Metformin

If the patient is type 2 diabetic and takes metformin, what important considerations are there?
The main concern is lactic acidosis.
The steps to take are
Withhold metformin for 48 hours after the IVU and restart if creatinine remains normal
If there is renal impairment, withhold metformin for 48 hours prior to the study.
If there is renal impairment and patient still takes metformin, keep patient well hydrated and stop metformin. Discuss with endocrinologist the need to change metformin long-term. **Iodinated contrast agents and renal impairment: (Both ionic and non-ionic contrast agents):**
If GFR <50 the physician will be notified.
If GFR <30 and the referring physician has determined that a contrast – enhanced imaging study must be done to obtain critical medical information, the contrast may be given after considering the following precautions:
Discuss the risks, benefits, and alternatives with the patient.
Adequate patient hydration must be maintained.
Optional treatments include the following:
N-acetylcysteine orally, 600 mg twice daily on the day before and the day of the contrast imaging study or
Bicarbonate 3ml/kg bolus, then 1ml/kg/hr x 6 hours (150 mEq in 1000 ml D5W

Common Urological procedures BAUS Consent forms

TRUS Prostate biopsies:
Common (greater than 1 in 10) (>10%)
Blood in your urine.
Blood in your semen for up to **6 weeks;** this poses no problem for you or your sexual partner.
Blood in your stools.
Urinary infection (10% risk).
Discomfort from the prostate due to bruising.
Haemorrhage (bleeding) making you unable to pass urine (2% risk).

Occasional (between 1 in 10 and 1 in 50) (2-10%)
Blood infection (septicaemia) needing admission (2% risk).
Haemorrhage (bleeding) needing admission (1% risk).
Failure to detect a significant cancer of the prostate.
The procedure may need to be repeated if the biopsies are inconclusive or your PSA level rises further.
Rare (less than 1 in 50) (<2%)
Inability to pass urine (retention of urine).
Hospital-acquired infection
Colonisation with MRSA (0.9% - 1 in 110).
MRSA bloodstream infection (0.02% - 1 in 5000).
Clostridium difficile bowel infection (0.01% - 1 in 10,000).
The rates for hospital-acquired infection may be greater in high-risk patients, for example those patients
with long-term drainage tubes;
who have had their bladder removed due to cancer;
who have had a long stay in hospital; or
who have been admitted to hospital many times.

Testicular Torsion consent
Common (greater than 1 in 10) (>10%)
Fixation of **both** testicles is usually required.
It may be necessary to remove the affected testis if it is too damaged to recover.
Occasional (between 1 in 10 and 1 in 50) (2-10%)
It may be possible to feel the stitch used to fix the testicles through the skin.
Blood collection around the testicles which resolves slowly or needs surgical removal.
Possible infection of the incision or the testis needing further treatment.
Rare (less than 1 in 50) (<2%)
Later shrinkage of the testicle, even if the testis is preserved.
No guarantee of fertility.

Hospital-acquired infection
Colonisation with MRSA (0.9% - 1 in 110).
MRSA bloodstream infection (0.02% - 1 in 5000).
Clostridium difficile bowel infection (0.01% - 1 in10,000).
The rates for hospital-acquired infection may be greater in high-risk patients, for example those patients
with long-term drainage tubes;

who have had their bladder removed due to cancer;
who have had a long stay in hospital; or
who have been admitted to hospital many times.

Vasectomy

Common (greater than 1 in 10)

A small amount of bruising and scrotal swelling for several days.

Seepage of a small amount of clear, yellow fluid several days later.

Blood in the semen for the first few ejaculations.

The procedure should be regarded as irreversible.

Although vasectomy may be reversed, this is not always effective in restoring fertility, especially if more than 7 years have lapsed since the vasectomy.

Sufficient specimens of semen must be produced after the operation until they have been shown to contain no motile sperms on two consecutive specimens.

Contraception must be continued until no motile sperms are present in two consecutive semen samples.

Chronic testicular pain (10 to 30%) or sperm granuloma (tender nodule at the site of surgery).

Occasional (between 1 in 10 and 1 in 50)

Significant bleeding or bruising needing further surgery.

Inflammation or infection of the testes or epididymis needing antibiotic treatment.

Rare (less than 1 in 50)

Early failure of the procedure to produce sterility (1 in 250 to 500).

Re-joining of vas ends, after negative sperm counts, resulting in fertility and pregnancy at a later stage (1 in 4000).

No evidence that vasectomy causes any long-term health risks (e.g. testicular cancer, prostate cancer).

Hospital-acquired infection

Colonisation with MRSA (0.9% - 1 in 110).

MRSA bloodstream infection (0.02% - 1 in 5000).

Clostridium difficile bowel infection (0.01% - 1 in 10,000).

The rates for hospital-acquired infection may be greater in high-risk patients, for example those patients
with long-term drainage tubes;
who have had their bladder removed due to cancer;
who have had a long stay in hospital; or
who have been admitted to hospital many times.

TURP

Common (greater than 1 in 10) (>10%)
Temporary mild burning, bleeding and frequency of urination after the procedure.
No semen is produced during an orgasm in approximately 75%. • Treatment may not stop all your symptoms. • Poor erections (impotence in approximately 14%). • Infection of the bladder, testicles or kidney which needs antibiotics. • Bleeding which may mean you have to go back to theatre or have a blood
transfusion (5%).
Possible need to repeat treatment later due to re-obstruction (approx 10%).
Injury to the urethra causing delayed scar formation.

Occasional (between 1 in 10 and 1 in 50) (2-10%)
Finding unsuspected cancer in the removed tissue which may need further treatment.
May need self catheterisation to empty bladder fully if the bladder is weak.
Failure to pass urine after surgery requiring a new catheter.
Loss of urinary control (incontinence) which may be temporary or permanent (2-4%).

Rare (less than 1 in 50) (<2%)
Irrigating fluids getting into the bloodstream, causing confusion and heart failure (TUR
syndrome).
Very rarely, perforation of the bladder requiring a temporary urinary catheter or open surgical
repair.

Hospital-acquired infection
Colonisation with MRSA (0.9% - 1 in 110).
MRSA bloodstream infection (0.02% - 1 in 5000).
Clostridium difficile bowel infection (0.01% - 1 in 10,000).
The rates for hospital-acquired infection may be greater in high-risk patients, for example those patients
with long-term drainage tubes;
who have had their bladder removed due to cancer;
who have had a long stay in hospital; or
who have been admitted to hospital many times.

Rigid cystoscopy
Common (greater than 1 in 10) (>10%)
Mild burning or bleeding on passing urine for a short period after the operation.
Temporary insertion of a catheter.
Occasional (between 1 in 10 and 1 in 50) (2-10%)
Infection of the bladder requiring antibiotics.
Finding of cancer or other abnormalities may require further surgery or other therapies.
Permission for telescopic removal/ biopsy of bladder abnormality/stone if found.
Rare (less than 1 in 50) (<2%)
Delayed bleeding requiring removal of clots or further surgery.
Injury to the urethra causing delayed scar formation.
Very rarely, perforation of the bladder requiring a temporary urinary catheter or open surgical repair.
Hospital-acquired infection
Colonisation with MRSA (0.9% - 1 in 110).
Clostridium difficile bowel infection (0.01% - 1 in 10,000).
MRSA bloodstream infection (0.02% - 1 in 5000).
The rates for hospital-acquired infection may be greater in high-risk patients, for example those patients
with long-term drainage tubes;
who have had their bladder removed due to cancer;
who have had a long stay in hospital; or
who have been admitted to hospital many times.

TURBT
Common (greater than 1 in 10) (>10%)
Mild burning or bleeding on passing urine for short period after operation.
Need for additional treatments to the bladder to prevent later recurrence of
tumours.
Occasional (between 1 in 10 and 1 in 50) (2-10%)
Infection of bladder needing antibiotics.
No guarantee of cancer cure by this operation alone.
Recurrence of the bladder tumour and/or incomplete
removal.
Rare (less than 1 in 50) (<2%)
Delayed bleeding needing removal of clots or further surgery.

Damage to drainage tubes from kidney (ureters) needing additional therapy.
Injury to the urethra causing delayed scar formation.
Perforation of the bladder needing a temporary urinary catheter or open surgical repair.
Hospital-acquired infection
Colonisation with MRSA (0.9% - 1 in 110).
MRSA bloodstream infection (0.02% - 1 in 5000).
Clostridium difficile bowel infection (0.01% - 1 in 10,000).
The rates for hospital-acquired infection may be greater in high-risk patients, for example those patients
with long-term drainage tubes;
who have had their bladder removed due to cancer;
who have had a long stay in hospital; or
who have been admitted to hospital many times.
Flexible cystoscopy

Common (greater than 1 in 10)
Mild burning or bleeding on passing urine for a short period after the operation.
Occasional (between 1 in 10 and 1 in 50)
Infection of the bladder requiring antibiotics.
Rare (less than 1 in 50)
Temporary insertion of a catheter.
Delayed bleeding requiring removal of clots or further surgery.
Injury to the urethra causing delayed scar formation.
Hospital-acquired infection
Colonisation with MRSA (0.9% - 1 in 110).
Clostridium difficile bowel infection (0.01% - 1 in 10,000).
MRSA bloodstream infection (0.02% - 1 in 5000).
The rates for hospital-acquired infection may be greater in high-risk patients, for example those patients
with long-term drainage tubes.
who have had their bladder removed due to cancer
who have had a long stay in hospital; or
who have been admitted to hospital many times

10. Appendix:
Comparison between the training route the CCT (National Training Number) NTN route and the non-training route CESR (Certificate of Eligibility for Specialist Registration) or previously article 14

Which route is better?

There is no right or wrong answer, both routes could lead to admission to the specialist register and the right to apply to consultant posts. It is more difficult to do so via the CESR route as the evidence required is more extensive and requires a lot of self-motivation, however it is not an impossible process and 50-60% of applications each year are indeed successful, especially if they start to collect evidence early on in the process (i.e. from day one). The CESR route is much more family friendly during the initial years compared to the NTN CCT route however the latter route becomes equally family friendly after finishing training and after the candidate becomes a consultant and works in the same hospital for the rest of his/her career. The quality of the job is perhaps slightly better in the NTN CCT route due to protected theatre time, however in the CESR route the doctor could be selective and choose a job that offers him his/her training needs matching that of the NTN CCT route. Many candidates taking the CESR route do not apply for consultant posts either because they choose to stay as specialty doctors due to family commitments or due to their reluctance to become a consultant and bear much higher level of responsibility for patient care.

	NTN CCT Route	**CESR/ Article 14 route**
Family life	Difficult, especially if married and have kids, Options include: 1- moving every year with the family to be near the hospital. 2- buy a house or have a base somewhere and either travel or rent next to the hospital if too far to travel. (Please note each deanery has allowance for renting/traveling expenses)* All these options are not ideal and quite disruptive to family life. Many trainees postpone marriage or having children until after finishing training for these reasons.	Easier, no need to travel you stay in the same hospital for 5-8 years until you achieve the required competencies and pass your FRCS Urol exam. You could buy a house near the hospital and you could see your family on a daily basis which is a privilege not to be underestimated.
Training	Generally well structured, Mostly deanery driven, you will have regular assessments (ARCP assessments on a yearly or six monthly basis) and regular teaching (on a monthly basis). You	Generally not very well structured. Mostly personally driven. You need to make sure your job provides you with adequate theatre exposure and enables you to fulfil the indicative numbers

		will have guaranteed theatre exposure, otherwise your deanery has the right to withdraw your post from the relevant hospital if you are not offered decent and sufficient theatre exposure. You have protected rights of training and the right to complain to your deanery if you don't get adequate training.	on your log book and perhaps develop a subspecialty interest if possible. You also need to complete lots of work based assessments (WBAs) and have evidence of everything you do. This requires a lot of self-motivation and drive on your part. On the other hand, if your job doesn't provide you with training opportunities and your consultant supervisors are not supportive, you need to discuss this with your consultants or consider quitting the job and find a better alternative if things are difficult to change.
Required evidence for the admission on the specialist register		You need to pass your annual ARCPs and collect enough WBAs. You need to have enough knowledge by passing the FRCS (Urol) exam and enough clinical experience covering a wide range of sub-specialties. Including paediatric urology. You also need to show evidence of operative	The evidence required is much more complicated and all need validation and authentication from supervising consultants. The doctor should have a clear plan from the beginning and get all the supervising consultants on board so that they could all

experience and competence. You need to show evidence of involvement in research (GCP certificate) and publication of two research papers in peer reviewed journals as first author. Also, you should have two presentations at national or regional meetings and complete a course in research methodologies. You should also do a quality improvement project. Attend 70% of the training sessions provided by the Deanery. Attend {Training the Trainers} course. Attend courses on management and leadership. Attendance at one international congress every two years.	work together to achieve the ultimate goal of gathering all the required evidence over 5-7 years and apply to be enrolled on the specialist register. It is divided into four domains: **First domain: Knowledge, Skills and performance.** This include qualification and certificates, assessments and appraisals. Passing the FRCS (Urol) exam. 360degree multi-source feedback, awards, personal development plans, logbooks, referral letters, rota, timetable and job plan. Evidence of research is very similar to CCT requirement (2 papers), presentation and poster presentation in national and international meetings. CPD points and records of attendances. Evidence of teaching and training, like teaching timetable

and evidence of feedback. **Second domain is safety and quality** like participation in audit and service improvement, reflective diaries, participation in clinical governance, attendance at appropriate courses for safety like infection control, safeguarding vulnerable adults, safeguarding vulnerable children, etc...**The third domain entails communication, partnership and teamwork**, this could be obtained from colleagues (multi-source feedback) and patients, participation in MDT, Management and leadership experience. This could be demonstrated by attending leadership and management training courses and appraisals which include this information. Charing meetings and leading projects. **Fourth**

			domain is called **maintaining trust** with evidence of honesty and integrity, like statements from referees and appraisal forms. Relationship with patients could be demonstrated with thank you letters, cards from colleagues and patients. Complaints and responses to complaints.
	Career aspirations	Vast majority of CCT trainees become urology consultants	Many Specialty doctors also apply for consultant posts but there are no accurate figures in the literature as to the percentage who applies. It seems to be around 30-40% or less whereas the rest stay in permanent non-training jobs (Many of whom out of choice, presumably to avoid moving and uprooting their families)
	Responsibility after finishing training	After becoming a consultant, you become the main responsible doctor for your own patient and consultants can deal with complaints and	Specialty doctors who don't apply for consultant posts as above have less responsibility as they will still be working under a named

	sometimes litigations.	consultant whom the bulk of the responsibility rests on his/her shoulders.
Sense of independence	Consultants are fairly independent and can have a say in their timetables etc…	Unless they become consultants themselves, Specialty doctors will always be under a consultant supervision and they might be asked to cover some duties often as a locum work in case of rota shortages, so they have less autonomy.
Quality of the job before and after finishing training	Before finishing training: good job quality, decent theatre exposure and teaching/training activities. After finishing training: tailored timetable and decent theatre time, good work-family balance.	Before finishing training: the quality of the job could be variable and the doctor is mainly responsible for accepting a job that offers him what he is after in terms of training and personal development. After finishing training: if the doctor become a consultant there is obviously no difference but if remains specialty doctor it depends on the doctor himself and his priorities the job might have less theatre exposure and contains more service element.

Table (8) Comparison between the CCT Route and CESR Route.
This link will explain the requirement for certification in Urology in the CCT route
http://www.jcst.org/quality-assurance/documents/certification-guidelines/CertificationguidelinesUrol2016FINAL.pdf
This link will explain the requirement for certification in Urology in the CESR non-training route.
http://www.gmc-uk.org/SGPC_SSG_Urology_DC2331.pdf_48455486.pdf

10.2. Invitation to interview letter

This is usually received via email upon successful longlisting for the interview. Please note that **there is no shortlisting for the interview**, i.e. if

ST3 Urology National Selection Interview Guide
Kass-Iliyya A.

you meet the essential criteria to apply for ST3 in Urology you will be longlisted and automatically receive an interview.

BEGINNING OF LETTER:
Invitation to Interview. National UROLOGY ST3 2016, 48 hour deadline.
Dear Sir/Madam
Re: Invitation to Interview: National UROLOGY ST3 2016, 48 hour deadline.
We are pleased to confirm that you have been invited to attend a **National Urology ST3 2016** Interview. The interviews will take place **on the 28th and 29th April 2016** at **Leeds United Football Club, Elland Road, Leeds, LS11 0ES.**
You should book a date and time slot for your interview on-line using 'Oriel'. You MUST login to your account within **48 hours (excluding weekends and Bank Holidays)** and respond whether you wish to ACCEPT or REJECT this invite. If you do not book by this time we will assume that you do not wish to attend the interview and your interview slot will be offered to another candidate.
To book your interview place, please log into your online account https://www.oriel.nhs.uk and enter your 'dashboard' then select the 'Interviews' tab at the top. Before booking your slot, please ensure you pay careful attention to any important details noted on the booking page; instructions on booking your interview are included in the 'Oriel' Applicant User Guide, which can be downloaded from https://www.oriel.nhs.uk
If you do not wish to attend the interview please let us know by formally withdrawing from the application process using 'Oriel'. We will then be able to offer your interview slot to another candidate. Please note that once you have formally withdrawn you will not be able to re-apply for this vacancy. Please note that this is a requirement set by the Department of Health and details can be found in section 5 of the Applicant Guide http://specialtytraining.hee.nhs.uk/specialty-recruitment/applicant-handbook/
Please arrive at the Interview reception no later than the start time you booked, we would also be very grateful if you do not arrive more than 30 minutes prior to this time.
PLEASE NOTE:- You will be at the interviews for approximately 3 hours from the time you book, this is essential to allow you to be registered, document checked and your portfolio to be analysed, then to conduct your interviews consisting of one 30 minute interview and four 15

minute Interviews (inc preparation time), and finally time for completing feedback and departure.

Water will be provided and there are a limited number of shops close by, however we advise candidates to bring additional food and refreshments as required.

ST3 Urology National Selection Interview Guide
Kass-Iliyya A.

You are required to bring Documents to the interview, these should be organised as outlined below, please ensure that original documents remain in your Portfolio.

1) Document Checking

There are a number of documents that you are required to bring for interview, these should be easily accessible and will be viewed alongside your original Documents (please ensure you have one copy of each original document on A4 paper only, with no paperclips, staples, plastic wallets etc) (your original Documents must remain in your portfolio). Please see the following link for a full list. You should check this list carefully; if you do not bring the correct documents you may not be interviewed.

1. Original passport plus one copy of the front cover, inside cover & signature/photograph page (originals plus 1 copy)
2. Original proof of address (original plus 1 copy)
3. Evidence of current immigration status i.e. original visa/Home Office documents, If on a Tier 2 visa please bring home office letter identifying your sponsor. (originals plus 1 copy)
4. GMC Certificate/Letter confirming receipt of annual retention fee/Letter confirming licence to practice/Proof of entry on the medical register (originals plus 1 copy)
5. Original primary qualification certificate (original plus 1 copy)
6. Evidence of core competencies, ie. ARCP CT2 with outcome 1 or "Urology Alternative certificate of core competence" (original plus 1 copy)
7. Evidence of English Language Competence if medical degree not taught in English, ie IELTS with score of 7 or more in each domain and an Overall score of 7.5 or more in a single sitting and within 24 months of the time of application, or letter from current clinical supervisor confirming satisfactory English Language skills for ST3 training (original plus 1 copy)
8. Evidence of completion of full MRCS (original plus 1 copy)
9. Portfolio and logbook (please see below)

You do not need to bring references to interview. References will only be requested for appointed candidates and these will be requested automatically by the Oriel system once an offer has been accepted.

2) Portfolio

You are required to bring your portfolio and associated logbooks to the interview, these will be collected after document checking. Your Portfolio will be reviewed and scored as part of a portfolio station and returned at the end of the interview process. Your portfolio should be clearly labelled and split into the following sections with an index at the front.

ST3 Urology National Selection Interview Guide
Kass-Iliyya A.

a) Degree certificates, Evidence of completion of MRCS, Foundation and Core competencies. Including Core training certificates with details of jobs undertaken for UK graduates and for others certificates of completion of posts from their trainers, programme directors or equivalent,
b) Course completion certificates,
c) Evidence of Prizes awarded.
d) Copies of the audits plus signed certification from trainers if presented or copy of journal / acceptance letter from journal if published,
e) Details and evidence of Teaching Experience
f) Copies of posters / presentations certified by trainers with details of where presented. Copies of Publications or letters of acceptance from peer reviewed journals for all publications.
g) Log book (this should not contain easily identifiable patient details other than unit number and date of birth or age)

Please note that hard copies of all documents are required as there is no internet access available at the interview venue.
Failure to produce documents or the falsification of documents, may lead to a referral to a scrutiny panel and / or disqualification from interview and GMC referral if appropriate.
For information and directions relating to the interview venue, please visit http://www.yorksandhumberdeanery.nhs.uk/recruitment/interviews/
The interview comprises of four 15 minute stations and one 30 minute station, these times include three-minute gap for movement and preparation between stations. Each station will be conducted by a group of assessors who will use the standardised scoring system.
The stations are

Portfolio / Career Progression – the portfolio will be inspected and assessed and you will be asked specific questions. Career progression involves a discussion about your previous training.
Clinical scenario (out patient) – an opportunity to explore your clinical management of the patient in an out-patient setting.
Clinical scenario (emergency) – a similar style, but in an emergency situation.
Communication – interaction with an actor simulating a patient or a relative.
Skills – this will test aspects of your technical ability.

ST3   Urology   National   Selection   Interview   Guide
                                                      Kass-Iliyya A.

Communication with other candidates regarding the content of the interview stations both during and after your interview is strictly forbidden. You must not take any notes about any aspect of the interview process or content away with you.

Interview expense claim details and forms are available from http://www.yorksandhumberdeanery.nhs.uk/recruitment/interviews/claiming_expenses_for_recruitment_(leeds_office)/

If you have any special needs for example in connection with a disability or your faith that you would like us to take into account in making arrangements for the interview, please make these known to urology.rec@yh.hee.nhs.uk with your "Surname, Forename" in the title of the email.

"By allowing applicants to progress to the interview stage, Health Education Yorkshire and the Humber HAS NOT accepted or confirmed that applicants meet all eligibility requirements. This includes immigration status, evidence of achievement of Foundation competencies or equivalent, and requisite length of time in training as per the relevant national person specification. This list is not exhaustive, and is applicable to all eligibility criteria. Applicants may still be withdrawn from the application process at any stage, including after the interviews have taken place, if the evidence pertaining to an eligibility criterion is found by Health Education Yorkshire and the Humber to be unsatisfactory."

If you need to make an enquiry please email urology.rec@yh.hee.nhs.uk with your "Surname, Forename" in the title of the email.

Notification of Terms to Applicants

Health Education Yorkshire and the Humber is currently seeking advice on whether it is classified as an Employment Agency for the purposes of the Employment Agencies Act 1973 ("the Act") and associated regulations. In the meantime, you are notified of the following terms and conditions that will apply to the provision of services by Health Education Yorkshire and the Humber in connection with the recruitment of junior doctors to training programmes.

1. The services provided include a work-finding service for which the Act prohibits Health Education Yorkshire and the Humber from charging a fee.
2. The services provided by Health Education Yorkshire and the Humber will be provided without any charge to either junior doctors or the NHS employers that engage them.
3. If it is determined that the Act applies to Health Education Yorkshire and the Humber, Health Education Yorkshire and the Humber will operate as an employment agency in providing the services.
4. Health Education Yorkshire and the Humber is authorised to act for NHS employers that are offering training posts as part of the junior doctor training programme and is not authorised to enter into contracts with junior doctors on behalf of those employers.

By proceeding with the application process you are deemed to accept these terms and conditions.

Yours sincerely

The Urology Recruitment Team

Health Education Yorkshire and the Humber

END OF LETTER

10.3. Route of application to the specialist register

It is worth mentioning that if you are successful in the national selection interview and before your national training number (NTN) can be issued the deanery needs to determine whether upon application to the Specialist Register you will apply through the CCT or CESR Combined Programme (CESR CP) route.

Trainees within the CCT route are appointed into GMC approved programmes at Foundation level and Core or Specialty Training level. On appointment they are issued with a NTN with a **suffix 'C'**.

Trainees appointed to CESR CP route would have undertaken a mixed programme of GMC approved posts (Core Training, LAT, FTSTA) and non-approved posts (Trust Doctor, LAS, Clinical Fellow) followed by appointment to a specialty specific training programme. On appointment to a specialty specific training programme, the post-holder is issued with a **suffix 'L'** which formally confirms that their existing portfolio and competency progression has been approved and will allow the post-holder to apply to the Specialist Register via Article 14. If you did not undertake educationally approved posts prior to your appointment, or cannot supply the required evidence that you did, then you will be allocated an NTN with **suffix "E"** to denote that, subject to your progress, when you complete your training programme, you will be eligible to apply to the GMC for a Certificate confirming Eligibility for Specialist Registration (CESR).

Trainees undertaking the CESR CP route or the CCT will have identical training in all aspects. CCTs and CESRs are different but equivalent routes to the Specialist Register. Having said that it's definitely worth getting a training number even if you get suffix L or E because your training will be easily recognised and validated via your ARCPs, which you can't guarantee easily with non-training posts. All these factors will make it much easier to make the CESR (CP)/CESR application with the help of the JCST who will recommend you to the GMC once the ARCP outcome 6 is signed off for the award of the CCT or CERS (CP) as appropriate. So basically whether you go through the CCT route or the CESR (CP)/CESR route the application is very similar. However, if you go through **the full CESR route** which you will choose if you obviously don't have a NTN and all your placements were in non-training posts, then the application is harder as you need to

validate all the evidence you provide and you need to rely on your own initiative to compile and authenticate the required evidence which is quite extensive but achievable if you plan early. See the following link
http://www.gmc-uk.org/SGPC__SSG__Urology__DC2331.pdf_48455486.pdf
For further information on different routes of specialty training and applying to be on the specialist register, please follow this very useful link which includes the Gold guide for higher surgical training.
http://www.jcst.org/archive/docs/gold-guides/gold-guide-2014
Please note that trainees with certification dates on or after the 1st of June 2016 will follow a new JCST certification process as per the following:
Certification dates from June 2016 onwards

Below is a description of the JCST's certification process for trainees with certification dates on or after 1 June 2016. We hope it will help you when your certification date approaches.
The new process has the support of both the Conference of Postgraduate Medical Deans (COPMeD) and the Confederation of Postgraduate Schools of Surgery (CoPSS).
JCST Office
Check trainee's training details and ISCP account six months before certification date
Inform the GMC that trainee is due to finish training
Advise trainee, Training Programme Director (TPD) and SAC Liaison Member (LM) that they need to prepare for the final ARCP meeting

Trainee
Ensure that your training details are up-to-date
Ensure ISCP portfolio is up-to-date in advance of ARCP meeting (please remember that it is essential that assessors have enough time to assess all your evidence ahead of the panel meeting; failure to provide this evidence in a timely manner could lead to an Incomplete ARCP outcome – see Gold Guide (sections 7.40 – 7.48))
Ensure requirements of specialty's Curriculum and Certification Guidelines have been met and are demonstrated on ISCP
Ensure any information/documents requested by the JCST have been sent to the JCST office
Ensure completion of the GMC's certification process. Any questions should be directed to the GMC

Training Programme Director (TPD) and LETB/Deanery
Prepare for final ARCP meeting
Ensure those who need to attend, specifically the SAC LM, have been given enough notice to be able to attend meeting (at least eight weeks)
TPD to discuss trainee with SAC LM and agree final decision i.e. the award or otherwise of an ARCP outcome 6
TPD to sign off online ARCP 6 - ideally the form should not be signed more than four months before trainees' expected certification dates
LETB/Deanery to sign off online ARCP 6

SAC Liaison Member (LM)
Review trainee's ISCP portfolio using specialty's Curriculum requirements, Certification Guidelines, and Certification Checklist (if relevant)
Discuss and advise TPD on trainee's eligibility for the award of an ARCP 6 and consequent recommendation for the award of a CCT or CESR (CP)
Attend final ARCP meeting (if this is not possible then liaise with the JCST office)
Once signed off by TPD, record comments on relevant ARCP form in ISCP - even if comments do not support award of ARCP 6. (To do this please log in to your ISCP account, go to "My Trainees>ARCP Management", select the relevant trainee and go to the bottom of the page to "Sign Offs" to add your comment)
The new certification process will rely on data and evidence recorded entirely in ISCP. The role of the SAC in recommending you to the GMC for the award of a CCT or a CESR (CP) is a major part of this process. This will however only be possible if SAC LMs are able to assess your competences as evidenced by the data you have recorded in ISCP in advance of your final ARCP meeting.

Subject to a number of final checks, once the ARCP 6 is signed off by all relevant parties, including the SAC LM, we will recommend you to the GMC for the award of the CCT or the CESR (CP) (as appropriate).

Please note that the sign-off on an ARCP 6 does not automatically lead to a recommendation to the GMC. The JCST office will ensure that all items mentioned above have been addressed before proceeding with the recommendation.

Please be aware that if you apply for your certificate more than six months after your certification date, the GMC may ask you to supply extra evidence of your professional activities since your completion date before awarding you your certificate.

The GMC has stipulated that all applications for certification must be made within 12 months of expected certification dates. If you do not submit your application for your CCT or CESR (CP) via GMC Online within this timeframe, you may need to apply via the full Certificate of Eligibility for Specialist Registration (CESR) route - please note that full CESR applications are assessed against the most up-to-date version of your specialty's curriculum.

You must be on the GMC's Specialist Register before you can take up a substantive UK consultant appointment. You may however be interviewed for consultant posts before you are on the Specialist Register, provided the date of the interview is no more than six months prior to your expected certification date.

May I wish you the very best of luck as you continue in your journey in urology and thank you for reading.

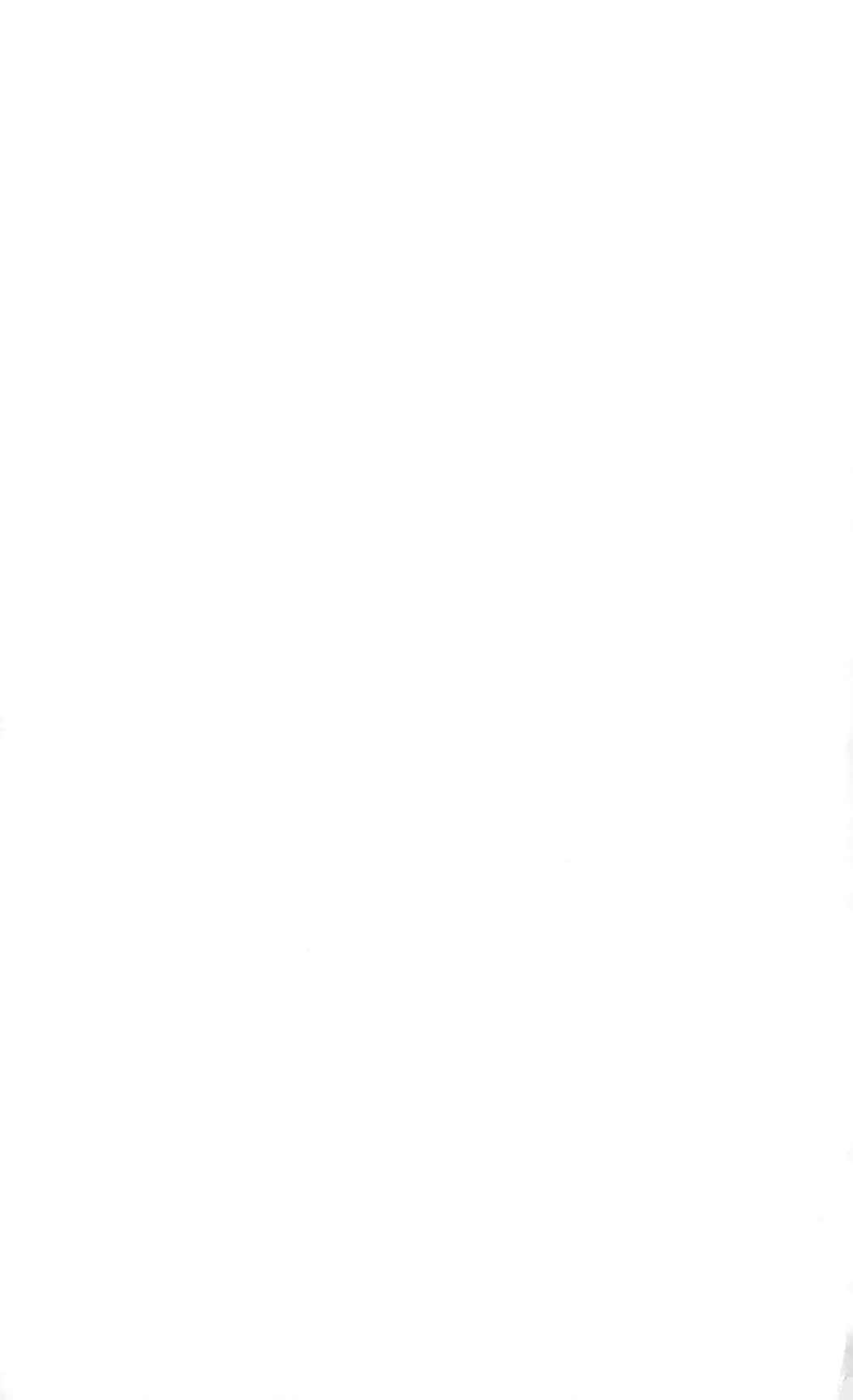

Printed in Great Britain
by Amazon